Oct. 19, 2020

M
I ho   njoy
del

dissecting your dreams
as much as I do.

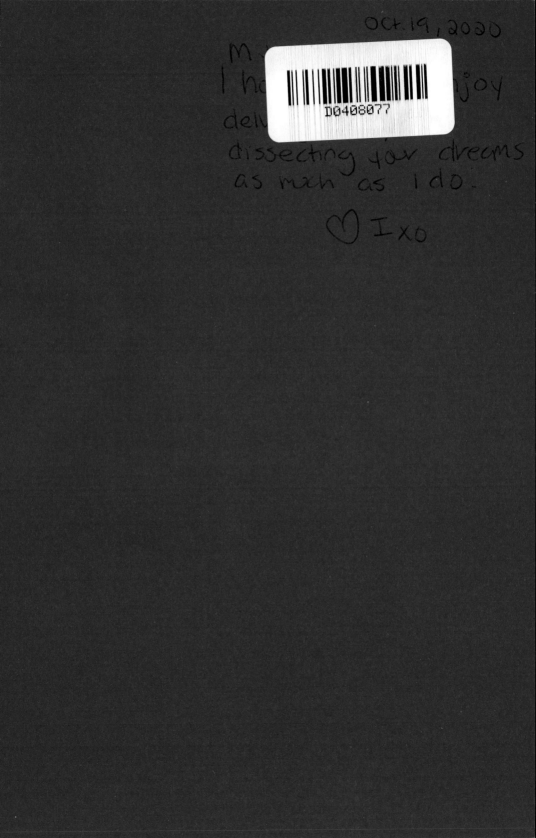 I xo

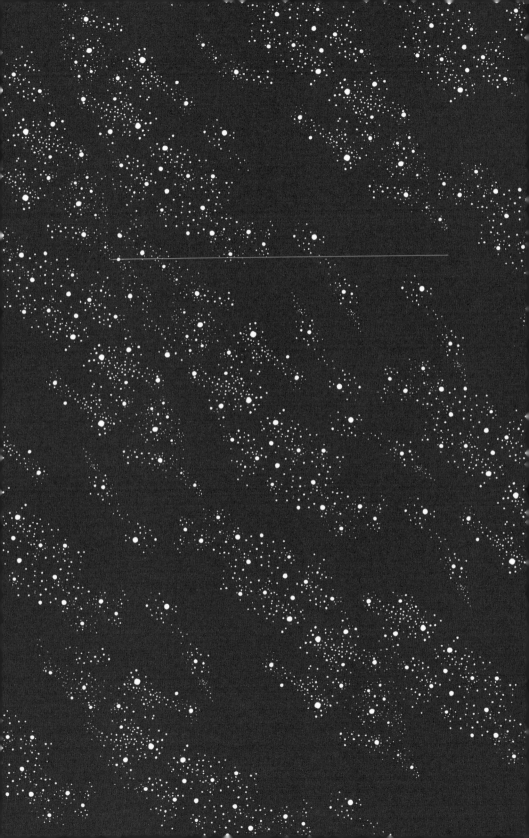

Text copyright © 2017 by BLACKIE BOOKS S.L.U.
Illustrations copyright © 2017 by Cristina Daura
Translation copyright © 2018 by Laura Ibáñez

Original idea and concept development: Blackie Books S.L.U.
Design by Setanta, www.setanta.es

Hachette Book Group supports the right to free expression
and the value of copyright. The purpose of copyright is to
encourage writers and artists to produce the creative works
that enrich our culture.

The scanning, uploading, and distribution of this book without
permission is a theft of the authors' intellectual property. If you
would like permission to use material from the book (other than
for review purposes), please contact permissions@hbgusa.com.
Thank you for your support of the authors' rights.

Voracious / Little, Brown and Company
Hachette Book Group
1290 Avenue of the Americas, New York, NY 10104
littlebrown.com

First North American Edition: October 2019

Originally published in Spain by Blackie Books S.L.U., 2017

Voracious is an imprint of Little, Brown and Company, a division
of Hachette Book Group, Inc. The Voracious name and logo are
trademarks of Hachette Book Group, Inc.

The publisher is not responsible for websites (or their content)
that are not owned by the publisher.

ISBN 978-0-316-53567-0
LCCN 2019937211

10 9 8 7 6 5 4 3 2 1

APS

Printed in China

THE BOOK OF

MY DREAMS

A JOURNEY TO SELF—DISCOVERY
AND CREATIVE FULFILLMENT

VORACIOUS

Little, Brown and Company

New York   Boston   London

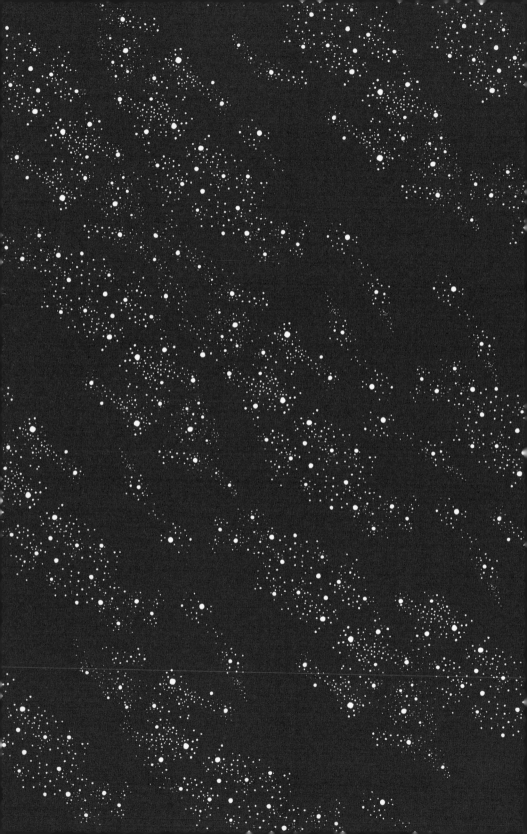

This book is a place to preserve your dreams. After all, it would be a shame to forget all those adventures.

With this diary, you can start exploring your memories and the journeys that your mind goes on at night.

It will inspire you and help you to understand yourself.

It will also be fun.

THIS IS THE BOOK OF
YOUR DREAMS

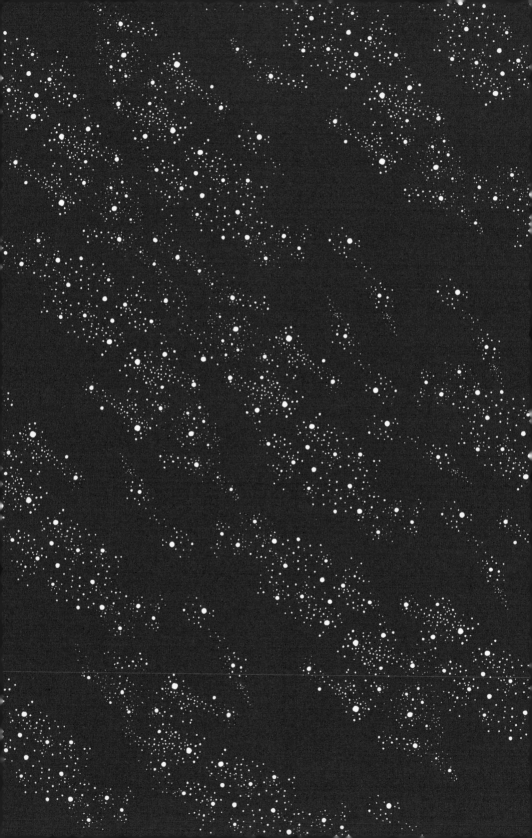

Personal Details

Name _____

Starting date of the diary _____

Age _____ How long do you sleep for? _____

Sleeping habits _____

Where do you usually sleep? _____

Between what hours? _____

How long does it take you to fall asleep? _____

With whom do you usually sleep? _____

Do you wake up at night?   Yes ◯ No ◯

Do you snore?   Yes ◯ No ◯

What's the best dream you can remember?
_____
_____
_____
_____
_____
_____

What's the worst nightmare you can remember?
_____
_____
_____
_____
_____
_____
_____

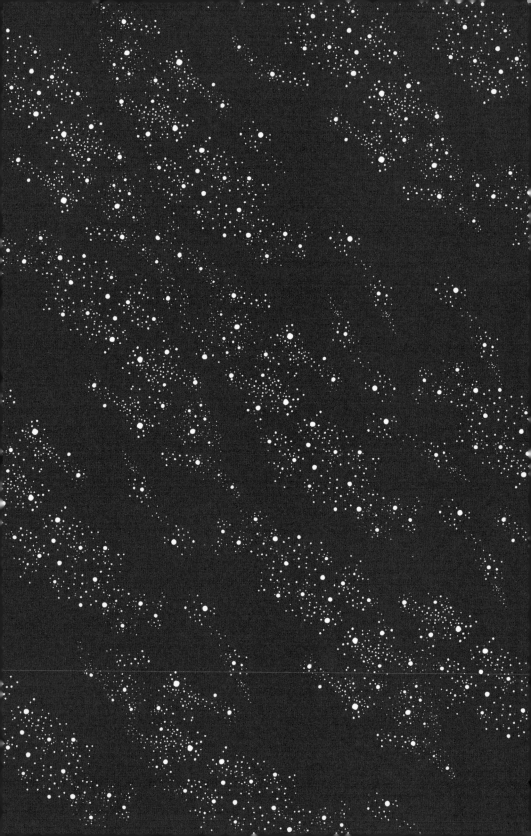

THE WORLD OF DREAMS

A brief history – scientific and practical – of the art of dreaming

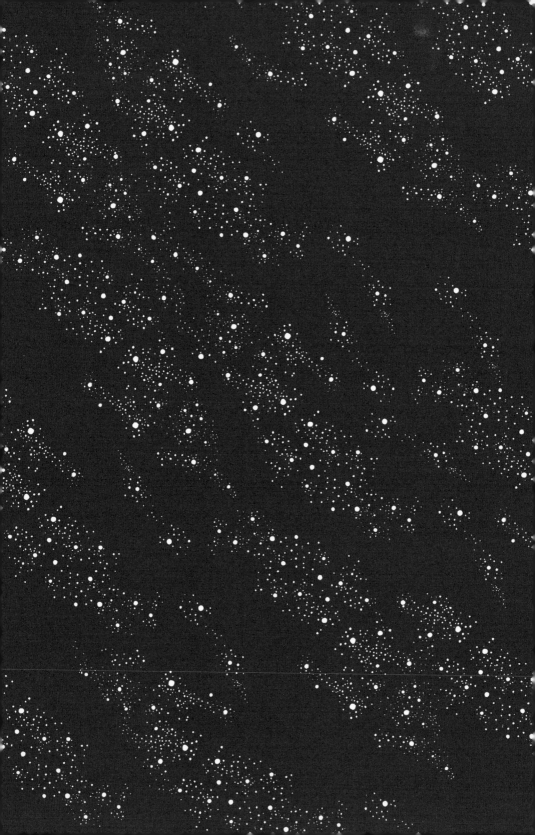

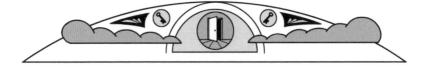

PROLOGUE

Our dreams are the diary of our lives: a place where our hopes, fears, desires and neuroses manifest as fantastical forms in stories ranging from the heartbreaking to the hilarious. In our dreams, we're all film-makers and novelists. Every night, we traverse secret, private worlds, built from the swirling undercurrents of our lives, yet we rarely pause to wonder why.

Could these dreams be maps to things we want for the future? Ways of healing past wounds? Attempts to make sense of the present?

Native Americans share their dreams every morning, picking them apart in search of moral guidance. When Charlotte Brontë wanted to write about something she hadn't experienced, she willed herself into dreaming about it first. The special theory of relativity, the sewing machine, benzene and various other scientific breakthroughs have all come about through insights gleaned from dreams. In fact, the basis for the entire scientific method we use today came to René Descartes in a dream involving ghosts, whirlwinds and a melon.

Still, most of us pay dreams little attention. Maybe the weirdest will be recounted to a bored friend, while they nod blankly and look left and right for escape routes. Maybe once a year you'll wake up feeling quietly aroused and vaguely guilty. And maybe a few will wake you at 4 a.m., with sweat rolling off your face and the terrified need for a hug pounding in your chest. Most though, will be irretrievably lost.

But what if we could get better at remembering them, so that almost no morning would go by without an exhilarating adventure to recall and deconstruct? And what if we could learn from these adventures? What if we could use them to gain a better understanding of ourselves? What if we could use them as fuel for creativity? And what if we could learn to wake up inside our dreams? To steer them in whatever direction we wanted?

This book aims to provide a place for you to learn and hone all of these practices. It's a secret diary laid out so that dreams can be easily catalogued and interpreted. After an introduction to various dreaming aids and practices, this book will be turned over to you. It will be yours to fill as you become more engaged and involved with the incredible experiences that unfold within you every night.

Let's stop missing out on a third of our lives. Let's start remembering. Let's dream.

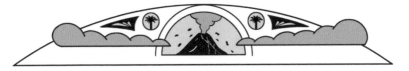

THE SCIENCE OF SLEEP

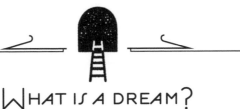

WHAT IS A DREAM?

ead down on the pillow, duvet pulled up over your shoulders, you close your eyes and wait. Some nights you go out like a light, others you lie for what feels like hours, tossing and turning while your brain wrestles with the anxieties and emotions of the day.

Eventually though, sleep comes.

You'll enter **stage one** sleep first, with the heart rate slowing and breathing becoming more regular. Any sounds might be noticed but you probably won't respond. You won't want to; you'll be drifting away from the waking world. This might feel like falling or glowing or fading out. There may be twitches or jerks as the body is slowly turned off. On average, this stage takes up around 5 per cent of the total sleep time.

After around ten minutes, **stage two** will begin. This is the first real period of sleep. The heart rate slows, breathing deepens, and the outside world is pushed even further away. Short, sharp bursts of brain activity serve to protect and maintain your sleep, while playing a key role in processing memory.

Stage two sleep is where you'll spend most of the night. You'll come back to this stage repeatedly over the course of an evening, spending around 50 per cent of the time here.

 Dreams that take place during REM sleep tend to feature small casts of familiar people, while those happening in non-REM more often have larger groups of less familiar characters.

Next comes **deep sleep**. Brain activity, breathing rate and heart rate are all at their lowest. The outside world is almost completely blocked out. This is the dark of the night. This is where nightmares, sleepwalking and sleep-talking are most likely to occur. Dreaming is a possibility here, although it's more likely to happen in the next stage. Deep sleep will make up around 20 per cent of the night.

Finally you enter rapid eye movement sleep, or **REM sleep**. Brain activity returns to levels similar to waking. Oxygen consumption, heart rate and blood pressure all climb back to near waking levels. Your eyes start to flicker back and forth beneath their lids while all other muscles are completely paralysed, a defence mechanism that keeps you from acting out the bizarre stories playing out in your head.

Though taking up only around 25 per cent of the night, this is where the majority of dreams take place.

Bizarre collages of thoughts and feelings, people and places, stories and situations: dreams are almost impossible to define but, for most of us, they need no introduction.

You're conscious again, but you're not in the world. Not the waking world anyway. You're receiving no sensory input. Every sight, smell, taste and texture is being generated by your brain. The world you're participating in exists only within yourself but, while it's happening, you don't know that. This purple planet is real, as are the monsters populating it, and the emotions that the situation provokes in you.

The logic centre of your brain has shut down while the emotional control core is hyperactive. You're not bound by what's real, you're living in a place built from thoughts and feelings. Instead of concrete language and realistic images, you're surrounded by symbols and abstract creations, wild manifestations of desires, fears, anxieties and memories.

These are dreams.

Maybe you'll remember them, maybe you won't. Maybe they'll be terrifying, maybe they'll soothe you. What is almost certain is that they will happen. Every night, seven or eight dreams will unfold within your brain as you sleep, and, by the end of your life, you will

 After the REM phase, the cycle begins again. It takes about ninety minutes from the beginning of the dream to the end of the REM episode.

have spent around six years dreaming. That's 2,200 days spent lost in worlds of your own creation.

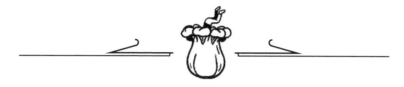

Why do we dream?

'We dream – it is good we are dreaming –
It would hurt us – were we awake –
But since it is playing – kill us,
And we are playing – shriek –'
'We dream – it is good we are dreaming',
Emily Dickinson

There are a vast number of different theories about why we dream. As is most often the case, it seems that each approach can provide us with a different piece of the puzzle. We're far from understanding the human brain, which puts us even further from understanding dreams, but we can say fairly surely: they happen for a reason. Dreams aren't plucked from nowhere and they aren't without their effects. Let's explore a few possible explanations.

EMOTIONAL STABILIZATION

Dreams are often likened to a kind of therapy. They take our emotions and give them shape, organize them into stories and present them to us in unexpected ways. Life is so relentless and overwhelming that dreams can be the alone time we need to spend reflecting and making sense of hectic days and their events.

We tend to dream in metaphors. Teeth fall out, waves crash over our heads and lions parade through our kitchens. They're not just replays of our memories, they're replays of emotions we've experienced through those memories.

The effect of these metaphors is to put abstract concepts in concrete terms. Freedom is a vague idea, while the feeling of flying is a tangible one. Anxiety is difficult to convey, while losing all your teeth is an easily understood experience. In this way, dreams can give clearer forms to complex emotional states. They can help us to process things by working through them from different angles and by building familiarity with the least familiar aspects of ourselves.

If you get robbed, for example, you're likely to dream of being robbed in the immediate aftermath of the event. After that, the dreams will probably become more symbolic, so that you might dream of being naked and vulnerable on a stage, or afraid and lost in a strange neighbourhood. Past that, the experience will have been fixed into your psychological landscape, and dreams will return to normal. The traumatic event has been revisited, reinterpreted and processed.

WISH FULFILMENT

Sigmund Freud was the first to suggest that dreams may simply be wish fulfilment fantasies. He claimed that our dreams take the form of our subconscious desires. You might dream of winning the lottery, becoming a successful writer or sleeping with a favourite celebrity.

Why? According to Freud, for the simple pleasure of it. In dreams, we can experience things that would otherwise be impossible, and in doing so we can gain a certain level of satisfaction.

Carl Jung offered a slightly different explanation. He posited that dreams were generally 'compensatory', meaning that the dreamer was conjuring those things they'd been denied. If they'd gone a while without sex, they might have sexual dreams, and if they were on a diet, they might dream of gorging themselves on crisps and chocolate cake. The subconscious is seeking to make up for what it misses out on during the day. Instead of desire, the focus is basic need.

Although you might be able to identify some dreams as being obvious wish fulfilment fantasies or compensations, these will represent only a small number of your dreams. It's impossible to fit all dreams into such narrow categories.

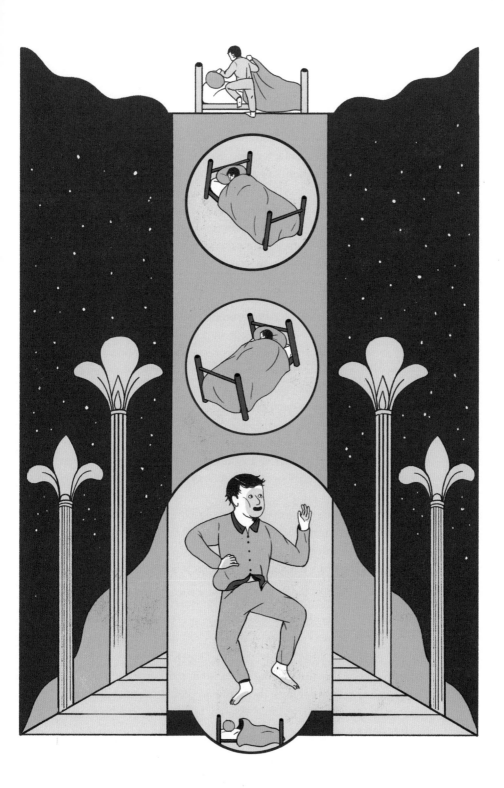

Every day, we take in huge amounts of information from the world around us. Most of it is useless and only a small fraction is retained in our long-term memories.

Strangely, it seems increasingly likely that dreams play a vital role in consolidating and storing memories.

One 2010 Harvard study saw ninety-nine volunteers attempting to memorize a 3D maze so that five hours later, when they were dropped at a random point in it, they'd be able to make their way as quickly as possible to a landmark. Half were allowed to nap during the five hours while the other half were kept awake. Amazingly, those that slept performed around ten times better on the task than those who didn't.

This might be explained by something called continual-activation theory, devised by the neurologist Jie Zhang. Zhang suggests that while we're awake, the memories we form aren't added directly to our long-term memories, but are instead kept in a kind of temporary folder. As we dream, these memories are processed and consolidated, and it is then that they're moved over into long-term storage. According to Zhang, dreams aren't the cause of this memory transference, just a phenomenon that results from it.

One therapeutic strategy arising from this idea has been to prevent victims of trauma from going to sleep for a period after they've experienced an ordeal, thus keeping the emotional memory from being so fully retained. Whether or not it's a healthy coping mechanism is questionable.

Studies of people with diseases that inhibit dreams, or those on medications that suppress REM sleep, have shown little effect on behaviour but big effects on learning.

There's a clear link between the two, but whether it's a cause or a correlation remains to be seen.

EVOLUTION

From an evolutionary perspective, it's possible that dreams are a means of rehearsing various threatening scenarios in a risk-free environment. The more we practise things, the better we get at them, and dreams might have provided a training ground for evading predators and hunting down prey.

Although the distance between us and our hunter-gatherer ancestors might mean our dreams are hugely different, if we observe how our pets behave while dreaming, we can see familiar behaviour. Most often, they appear to be chasing prey, perhaps as a form of practice. Maybe this is how our own dreams started out.

Another evolutionary theory is based around similarities between animals that are playing dead and humans who are dreaming. The dreaming brain is nearly as active as the waking brain, with the crucial difference being that the body is paralysed, which means that dreams may be the remnants of a defence mechanism in which we once deterred predators by pretending to be dead.

There are a number of theories as to why we dream but perhaps they're not as important as what we can get out of dreaming. They may be an evolutionary adaptation, they may be chance happenings, but that doesn't mean they can't provide us with insight and inspiration if we take the time to look.

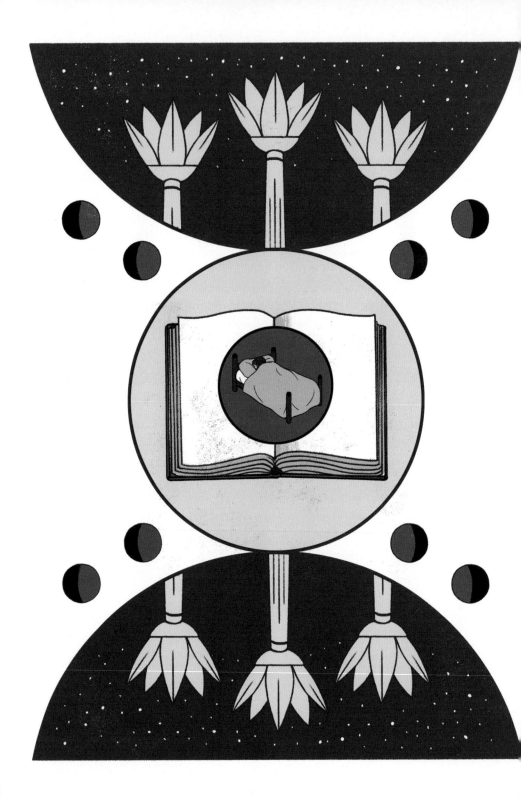

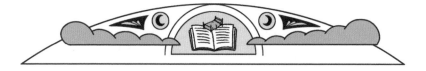

A FIELD GUIDE
TO DREAMING

SLEEP HYGIENE

First things first: to dream, we have to sleep. The majority of people don't get enough sleep and the sleep they do get tends to be restless and unsettled. Why? It's generally down to poor sleep hygiene caused by our bodies struggling to make sense of the modern world. From bright lights in the night-time to dim offices in the day, we are constantly confusing the clocks that control the cells of our bodies.

Sleep is regulated by circadian rhythms, which are how the cells of our bodies know when to perform activities like dividing, regenerating, producing hormones, and almost everything else you can think of. Every single cell in your body, from your toenails to your lungs, has its own circadian clock, and these clocks are tied to the passing of days and nights. As the sun sets, a chemical called melatonin is

A study of over 10,000 British civil servants carried out over five years showed that those who reduced their average sleep from seven to five hours had a 70 per cent increased risk of mortality from all causes. Those who slept more than eight hours also had double the risk of mortality, mostly from non-cardiovascular causes.

The conclusion? We should be aiming for around seven hours of sleep a night.

released into the cells, letting them know it's time for bed; then, as the sun rises, the production of melatonin drops off and the cells alter their actions accordingly.

Modern habits are out of sync with the natural circadian rhythms of our bodies. Instead of sunlight in the daytime and darkness and night, we sit indoors during the day and surround ourselves with light bulbs, laptops and TVs in the night hours. The main problem with electronic devices is that they emit blue light, which suppresses the release of melatonin more than light of any other kind, meaning that cells aren't receiving the news that the time for sleep has come.

The human sleep cycle has evolved over thousands of generations, and deviation from it has consequences not just for sleep and dreams but for our health and mortality. Studies of shift workers have shown them to be at increased risk of cancer, obesity and a litany of other ailments. There's almost no cell in the body that isn't affected by sleep.

Despite it being near impossible to revert to the way our ancestors slept, there are a number of changes that can be made to improve our quality of sleep:

• Total darkness in the bedroom, for obvious reasons. If you find this hard to achieve, think about trying a sleeping mask.

• Use your bedroom only for sleep and sex. While it's tempting to lounge around on the duvet in the day, it can lead to your brain linking being in bed to being mentally alert, making it harder to switch off when it's time to sleep.

• No computer or TV at least an hour before bed. If you absolutely have to work online, try downloading a program like F.lux which automatically switches your screen to an orangey colour in the evening, thus reducing the amount of blue light you're exposed to before bed.

• As little caffeine, nicotine, alcohol and other drugs as possible in the hours before bed. All are stimulants that decrease sleep quality and time spent in deep sleep.

• Cardiovascular exercise of even ten minutes can drastically improve sleep but it should take place at least three hours before bed.

• Exposure to daylight as soon as possible after waking and preferably at least an hour in direct sunlight during the day. If it's not possible, consider a cheap light therapy lamp, which will also come in useful during winter months.

• A consistent sleep pattern. Try to wake up at the same time and get to bed at the same time each day as it will help your circadian rhythm to function at its best.

It might seem overwhelming, but even small alterations in the way you sleep can have big repercussions for health and dreaming. By upping the quality and duration of your sleep, you'll find yourself learning more, remembering more, feeling happier, having more stable moods, falling ill less often, making mistakes less often and generally feeling better. You'll also find that as you start to sleep better, you start to dream better. And those dreams might be important.

 If, even after adjusting your sleeping environment and habits, you find it hard to catch a good night's sleep, you might want to visit your doctor or try experimenting with one of these natural sleeping aids:

• Melatonin supplements are taken an hour before bed and make up for the suppression of melatonin by blue light.

• Calcium is vital to sleep as it's used by the brain to turn tryptophan into melatonin. A glass of milk or kefir will keep you covered.

• Passionflower tea has been proven to be as effective as certain benzodiazepines for anxiety. If it's worry that's keeping you awake, this might help.

• Valerian root is another tea that's been shown to calm the nerve cells in the brain.

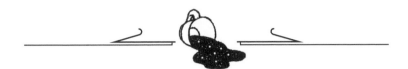

INPUTS AND OUTPUTS

Have you ever felt lazy after eating an entire pizza? Sleepy after steak? Fresh and ready for the day after a bowl of cereal topped with blueberries, yoghurt and almonds?

Different foods affect how we feel during our waking lives, so isn't it only natural they affect what happens in our dream lives?

The idea of the food we eat affecting the dreams our brains conjure at night can be traced as far back as Hippocrates, through Greek dream cults and Egyptian dream temples, right the way to recent studies about the effects of fast food on dreaming. Along the way, a number of myths regarding food and dreams have sprung up: cheese inducing nightmares, spicy foods giving rise to surreal dreams, and even Romantic poets consuming rotten meat in the hopes of more exciting nocturnal imaginings.

Almost all are probably false.

There's no proven link between cheese and nightmares; spicy food is more likely to lull you into dreamless sleep; and Romantic poets eating rotting meat would be more likely to wake up needing to vomit than transcribe their most recent nocturnal adventures.

Here is where we face a slight dilemma: if, before bed, you eat a

 One study, however, conducted by the British Cheese Board in 2005, did manage to find a strange correlation between consumption of cheese before bed and dreams. Out of 200 participants, 72 per cent reported sleeping very well and 67 per cent could recall their dreams, with the surprising result that amongst those 67 per cent, the eating of certain types of cheese seemed to cause different types of dreams.

Stilton: bizarre dreams.
Red Leicester: dreams of the past.
Lancashire: dreams of the future.
Cheddar: dreams about celebrities.
Cheshire: dreamless sleep.

heavy meal that's tough on your stomach, you will be more likely to wake up in the night, meaning you will be more likely to remember whatever dream you were engaged in. You won't, however, be particularly well rested, and the dreams you're remembering probably won't be particularly peaceful either.

Have you ever had a sound or smell clamber from the waking world into one of your dreams? Drilling on the street outside your house or the smell of bacon wafting through from the kitchen? If the sensory input you're receiving comes in the form of an upset stomach, it's unlikely to shape the most beautiful or calming of dreams.

Equally, an empty stomach may have adverse effects on the kind of dreams we experience. It's an extreme example, but some studies have shown that anorexics dream almost entirely about food. Our bodies, when deprived of something, often turn to dreams to make sense of this deprivation. It seems that the best solution is to go for a small snack before bedtime if needed, and ideally for a snack that contains a chemical called tryptophan.

 The neuroscientist Gary Wenk recommends a peanut butter and jelly sandwich as the perfect pre-sleep snack. The bread will help get you to sleep, while the sugar provides fuel for a dreaming brain.

Tryptophan is found in a vast array of foods including nuts, poultry, red meat, fish, oats, beans and eggs. It's an amino acid that leads to the production of serotonin, which, along with melatonin, plays a key role in regulating our sleep cycles.

Carbohydrates help with getting tryptophan to the brain, which is part of the reason why meals consisting of heavy carbs can leave us feeling sleepy.

What about drinking? The idea of having a glass of whisky or wine before bed to get us off to sleep is a common one, and though it can help us to nod off faster, we tend to slip into less restorative, less deep and, crucially, less REM sleep after drinking. We also tend to recall fewer dreams in less detail while under the influence of alcohol.

And who wants to spend time scribbling into a dream diary while hung-over?

It's not all bad news though. If you have the possibility of sleeping in late the day after a drinking session, you may be able to reap the benefits of what's known as 'REM Rebound.' What this means is, if you've been prevented from achieving REM sleep previously, you'll slip into it far quicker than usual, leading to more vivid dreams in a shorter space of time.

Aside from pizza and beer, there's one substance that has been shown to alter not just the content of dreams, but our ability to recall them: vitamin B_6 is available to buy at chemists and health food shops, and a dose of between 100mg and 250mg, taken around an hour before bed, can lead to dreams of unbelievable intensity, emotion and vividness, apparently due to its effects on cortisol in the brain. In the interests of research, the authors of this book have experimented with the ingestion of vitamin B_6 before bed, and found its effects to be startling. Though it's too intense an experience to be repeated regularly, and overconsumption of B_6 could, in the long term, lead to side effects, you may want to consider this as a one-off investigation into what your brain is capable of.

Essentially, there are pros and cons in terms of dreaming to almost anything you ingest before bed. Some foods may help you into deeper sleep, while some will rouse you in the middle of the night, with dreams still fresh in your mind. After a few weeks of keeping a diary, you'll find yourself naturally remembering more dreams regardless. The ability to recall dreams is like a muscle that needs training: the more you practise, the more you'll remember.

Try logging what you eat or drink before sleep and seeing if there's any correlation to your own dreams. You might be surprised by the results.

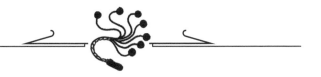

LUCID DREAMING

You're being pursued through an unfamiliar city by hordes of lizard-men. You're standing in a field of poppies, frantically trying to catch your own teeth as they tumble from your mouth. You're naked, sweating and clutching a violin in front of a baying audience of thousands.

Wait a second, you think. There's something strange about this. This doesn't make sense. Why am I here?

Cautiously, you jump, expecting a second in the air followed by a dull thump as you land back on the ground. But no thump comes. You look down, seeing the earth a few feet under you. Am I floating?

I'm dreaming, you realize.

And with that realization, you become the ruler of this bizarre kingdom.

You're no longer a passive player, being chased and trapped and led in circles, you're now in control. The lizard-men become puppies, your teeth are butterflies, and that useless violin is a rocket that will carry you up into the sky. You can fly over oceans, trek through the jungles of Peru or wander idly through an English village. You could access your unconscious, engage in sexual experiences or meet your heroes. You might even twist your nightmares into manageable forms, beating them into submission.

You've realized you're in a dream and now you're lucid dreaming.

The practice of learning to become aware while within a dream is another that dates back to ancient times. Greeks, Indian Hindus and Tibetan Buddhists all had their own methods of achieving such states. From meditation to drugs, yoga to unusual sleeping positions, people have long sought out ways to seize control of their dreams.

More modern practitioners of lucid dreaming are called oneironauts. They meet in conferences across the globe to lecture, discuss and trade information regarding ways and means of accessing and engaging with the dream world. One of the foremost modern oneironauts is a scientist named Stephen LaBerge, founder of the Lucidity Institute.

LaBerge carried out a number of studies wherein participants apparently in the midst of REM sleep would perform predetermined eye movements to prove themselves aware. Both these, and the testimonies of hundreds of thousands of oneironauts, point towards the phenomenon of lucid dreaming being a very real one. LaBerge goes so far as to claim that in a few decades' time, we'll all be routinely engaging in it, using it as a tool for overcoming anxieties, exploring ourselves and simply having enjoyable experiences.

While you may have inadvertently experienced one or two lucid dreams, it's unlikely you feel you have any control over when they might happen. But they're not random happenings. With a little practice, not only can the likelihood of lucid dreaming increase, but the scope of what you stand to gain from this practice can be multiplied.

There are a number of differing modern methods for inducing lucid dreaming, and here we'll focus on an amalgam of the most common, including both preparatory measures and steps to take immediately before and during sleep. It's not necessary to follow every step constantly; these are only suggestions, and it's possible that adding even a single one to your routine may be enough to begin your adventures in the world of lucid dreaming.

PREPARATIONS

Improve Your Sleep Hygiene

If we sleep well, we dream well. To enter long, undisturbed periods of REM sleep is increasingly difficult, but we only dream during REM so we want our REM sleep to be as sustained as possible.

Maintain This Dream Diary

Getting into the habit of noting down your dreams will naturally lead you to become more aware of them. You'll start paying them more attention, not just consciously but subconsciously, so that even as they unfold you'll be mentally taking notes.

Recognize Recurrences

If you've been keeping this dream diary filled with your experiences,

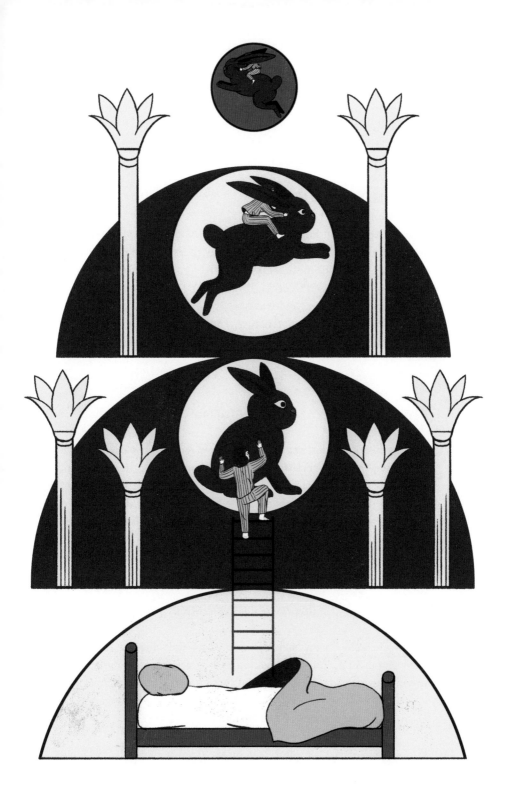

you may begin to see recurring themes and motifs. Once you see a common trope, it can often be enough to trigger a lucid dream.

Other reality checks: try the light switches. Read a clock. Look at your own reflection. Jump.

Practise Reality Checks

Reality checks are the foundations of lucid dreaming. They are a series of tests carried out, both while awake and while asleep, to help the oneironaut ascertain whether or not they're in the waking world or the dream world. The most common involves pushing the finger of one hand into the palm of the other. If the finger sinks through the palm, you're dreaming. If not, you're awake. Practise it around twenty times a day, until it becomes second nature. There are also a number of other reality checks that may be employed in addition to this one.

FIVE STEPS TO A LUCID DREAM

Step One: Meditate

This may seem a daunting prospect, but even ten minutes of meditation before bed can help calm the restless mind, increasing the chances of gaining awareness while you're in a dream. There are a number of free guided meditation apps available, but simple breathing-focused exercises will do just as well. Try focusing on the sensation of your breath as it enters your nostrils, and again as it exits. Allow thoughts to come and go, to drift past like clouds, but always return your attention to the sensation of air moving through you.

Step Two: Recite Mantras

Wanting to lucid-dream can play a large part in inducing one. As you fall asleep, try mentally uttering a mantra such as 'I am about to dream' or 'I am going to lucid-dream now', thus priming yourself for what's to come.

Step Three: Wake Up and Get Back Down

This is one of the simplest and most effective methods for lucid dreaming. It simply involves waking up for twenty to forty minutes around six hours after you've gone to bed. Spend the time thinking, jotting down dreams or reading a book, and once you return to sleep, your chances of entering a lucid dream will be tripled. The technique works because you're engaging your conscious brain at a time when it was expecting to be in the midst of REM sleep. After a few attempts, you may find they'll overlap, and you'll be plunged into a lucid dream.

Step Four: Engage Reality Checks

If you've been practising reality checks during the daytime, they should start to come naturally to you in dreams. Once that finger sinks through your palm, you'll know which world you're in.

Step Five: Go!

Visit other planets, other ages, other species. Become an animal. Become a superhero. Live out your favourite novel. Meet anyone who ever existed, past or present, real or not. Hold a council of wise men to determine whether or not you should leave your job. Rehearse interviews for a new job. Play the harp. Have sex. Summon a storm.

Explain to someone that they're a character in your dream: they're not real, you made them up. Swim deep in the ocean. Sit alone on a forest floor. Lie down on the moon, admiring Planet Earth.

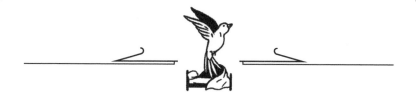

THERAPEUTIC DREAMING

B
oggarts are creatures in the Harry Potter universe that take the shape of whatever the observer fears the most. From petrifying creatures to deceased relatives, they're able to peer inside the hearts of wizards, identify what terrifies them most and adopt that form.

The only spell that can conquer them is the 'Riddikulus' charm.

What it entails, essentially, is turning the object of your fear into an object of ridicule using a feat of imagination.

When Neville saw Snape, he dressed him in his grandmother's clothes; when Padma saw a huge cobra, she transformed it into a jack-in-the-box; and when Ron was confronted with a giant spider, he made its legs disappear, so that it rolled uselessly on the floor like a raisin.

We can employ an almost identical tactic in lucid dreams. Once we've recognized that a nightmare is a nightmare, we can, using our imaginations, steer it away from the terrifying and towards the hilarious or absurd. LaBerge himself mentions meeting a seven-foot-tall barbarian in his dreams and defeating him by transforming him into a rainbow.

 In Guatemala and Mexico, small hand-made dolls are often given to children in times of emotional upheaval. The children tell these 'worry dolls' their fears and anxieties before bedtime then fall asleep with the dolls beneath their pillows in the hope that, by morning, the dolls will have taken their worries away.

The opportunity that lucid dreaming offers us is to confront our fears in a risk-free environment. That snake can't hurt you, the concert can't fail, and when you fall, you won't get hurt. Once we understand that, we can start using the dream world as a training ground for the waking world.

What about when we're faced with fears in non-lucid dreams? There are any number of ways that fears and anxieties can manifest themselves, but some of the most striking and consistent are in the dreams of recovering addicts. There are certain dreams that seem to crop up again and again for those in recovery, and the content of these dreams can tell us a lot about their possible functions. The three most reported are:

Dreams of Relapse

These are the most basic form of revelatory dream. The mind is wishing for something it used to have but no longer does, or something it never had but pines for nonetheless. Anorexics may dream of food, recovering addicts may dream of drugs, and the lonely might dream of company. It's your body's way of telling you what it wants, and whether or not it should get that is up to you.

Dreams of Going Back

These are dreams in which the addict is plunged back into the midst of their addiction. They've returned to the pits of despair and are again battling the demons they may have thought they fought off years previously. What's the use of this kind of dream? It may be a way of reminding the dreamer how bad things once were. Once you're along the road to recovery, it's easy to forget how life used to be, and to become complacent. These kinds of dreams offer both a reminder and a warning.

Dreams of Suicide

Death in dreams rarely relates to actual death. Generally, it signifies rebirth, growth and change. For the addict, it can be a sign that their recovery is on the right track and that they're starting to escape their former selves.

The feelings behind these three types of dreams are common to us all, as is the experience of having the subconscious reach out to the waking self. A dream of flight might let you know that your subconscious has finally given up on a lost love. A dream of being alone might remind you to keep your friends close. And a dream of running outdoors might mean your body is yearning for some kind of freedom.

There are times, though, when dreams might point towards something more straightforward: physical illness. It's generally accepted that there are detectable signs of sickness in most people before obvious symptoms arise, which means, basically, that our bodies know we're sick before we do. Is it so outlandish to think this could manifest in our dreams?

One woman dreamt her head was shaved with the word 'cancer' written on it, and, three weeks later, she was diagnosed with breast cancer. One man dreamt of Egypt after experiencing eye trouble there ten years previously, then, a few days later, his eye trouble started up again. There are numerous accounts of people having dreams featuring vampires biting at their necks going on to be diagnosed with thyroid problems. One Swedish study linked frequent nightmares in older people to heart trouble.

It may sound frightening, but more than anything, couldn't it be useful? What if paying attention to our dreams could get us to seek help sooner for problems that may worsen if left unchecked? By keeping a dream diary, you'll be able to notice any persistent or unusual dreams involving certain parts of the body. And that may just come in helpful.

Dreams can be beneficial to us in a vast array of ways, whether they're led by us or revealed to us. The key is to listen. In dreams, your subconscious will very often spell out what it wants, misses or needs. We are all multifaceted creatures, and often dreams are the only opportunity these different sides of ourselves have to meet.

We all live inner lives, voluntarily or involuntarily, and we can either choose to embrace and explore them or we can ignore them entirely. The risk, of course, is that if we ignore them, we ignore a potential source of valuable information about what's going on within us. Besides, ignoring something never made it go away.

Not only does lucid dreaming have potential benefits for overcoming our deepest fears, ideas have also been floated about its possible uses as a training tactic for various sports and disciplines.

Visualization has long been seen as a key tool in the arsenal of sportspeople, but it's only fairly recently that the degree to which it can improve performance has been realized. In one study, a group of basketball players were tested on how many free throws they could make, and then split randomly into three groups.

For a month, the first group practised an hour on court per day, the second group visualized themselves making free throws for an hour a day and the third group did nothing. The results were incredible. The first group improved by 24 per cent, the third group didn't improve at all, but the second group improved by 23 per cent.

And aren't lucid dreams the perfect playground for sports practice? Aren't they a risk-free environment in which we can run, leap and fall? Why stop there? Why not populate your dreams with German-speaking characters as you try to learn the language? Or spend dream-time practising Bach sonatas on a flute?

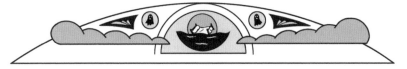

WHEN SLEEP
GOES WRONG

We all experience problems with sleep at some point in our lives: not enough of it, too much of it, nightmares, mumblings, nocturnal fights with imaginary beings. Most sleep disruptions are temporary, happening after long journeys or emotional days, but in some instances people suffer from chronic conditions that severely impact their waking lives. In these cases, not only can dreams turn dark, they may converge with reality in potentially dangerous ways.

From insomnia to narcolepsy, sleep apnoea to somniphobia, there is a vast array of disorders affecting sleep. Let's have a look at three that have special relevance to dreaming.

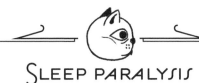

SLEEP PARALYSIS

Your eyes flick open. You're in bed. You can't move.

There are noises. A hammering at the door? Breathing in your ear? Cackling?

Shapes shift at the edges of your vision and shadow people loom from the corners of your room. There's someone in here. Something. And it's advancing.

You struggle with your body, willing it to move. It stubbornly refuses. Not even your toes respond. You can't breathe and it's as though a great weight's pushing down on your chest. You try to open your mouth and cry for help: nothing.

How long does this go on? Seconds? Minutes? It's impossible to tell. It's terrifying and it feels like you're going to die. But you don't. You never do.

Gradually, you regain control of your body and rejoin the world. You're safe.

One of the most commonly experienced dream phenomena is called sleep paralysis. Though it's estimated that up to 50 per cent of people will experience at least one episode in their lives, they tend to either be forgotten or get shrugged off as unusually vivid nightmares.

Attacks take place either as sufferers are falling asleep or as they're waking up, and they occur when sleep states overlap. While the body remains paralysed to keep you from acting out your dreams, the mind becomes alert and ready to enter a waking state. Though they've never been fatal, attacks of sleep paralysis can often feel life-threatening.

Sleep paralysis is most common for younger people and people with mental illness, though there's also a genetic component, and times of severe stress can also induce attacks. What sufferers experience can range from mild discomfort through to full-blown hallucinations.

Culture plays a part in what and whether sufferers are likely to hallucinate. In Germany, a small demon in a hat is liable to position itself on your chest. If you're in Italy, you might be set upon by a witch or a crazed cat. Aliens are often blamed for instances of sleep paralysis in America. While in Egypt, it's believed that the jinn, or evil genies, are responsible.

Interestingly, Egypt also has a far higher number of people reporting sleep paralysis in general, with three times as many sufferers as in Denmark. This is most probably down to having such a developed set of beliefs around the phenomenon, compared to Denmark, where it passes fairly unacknowledged.

So what we experience may hinge on what we expect to experience, and this can be true not just of nightmares but also of our

 How can you cope with attacks of sleep paralysis? A technique called meditation–relaxation therapy is suggested for those in the midst of an attack. It involves four simple stages. **1.** Keep your eyes closed and remind yourself that this is a biological happening, not a supernatural one. **2.** Remember that this is not an unusual occurrence and that it's impossible for any harm to come to you. **3.** Choose a happy memory and dwell on it. Bring it to life inside your head. Turn your attention inward. **4.** While focusing on the memory, don't make any attempt to move or to take control of your breathing.

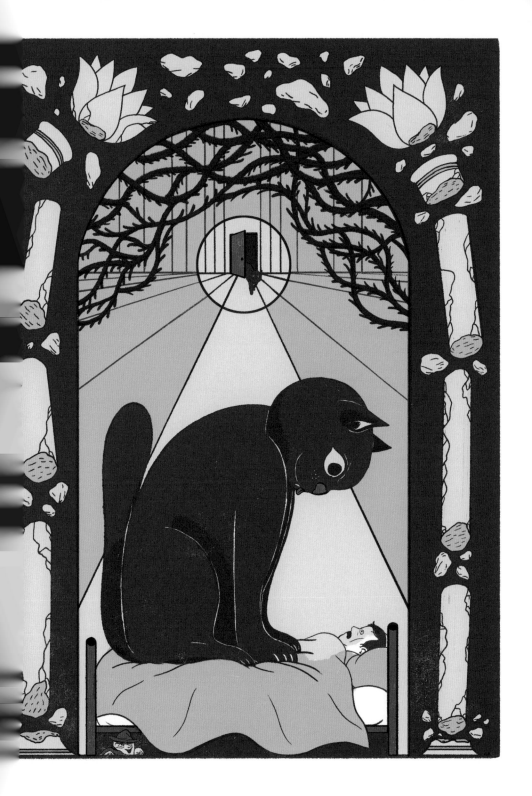

less foreboding dreams. If we expect to dream, we may be more likely to. And if we expect to remember those dreams, we may be more likely to do that too.

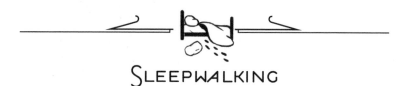

SLEEPWALKING

Sleepwalking is a disorder belonging to a group called parasomnias, which includes teeth grinding, sleep eating, sleep sex and exploding head syndrome. It involves a sufferer performing complex behaviours while asleep, generally something more than just walking. If the sufferer is dreaming, these may be related to the dream. If not, they may be mundane activities such as washing dishes, getting dressed or brushing their teeth. In some cases, the sufferer may go on long jaunts or drives.

Most often, though, sleepwalkers seem to perform bizarre, nonsensical actions, such as urinating in cupboards, pacing around rooms and clambering over furniture. Their eyes will be glassy, their faces blank and their talking incomprehensible. For onlookers, the experience can often be frightening.

The idea that it's dangerous for a sleepwalker to be woken is a

 One of the most notorious cases of sleepwalking involved a French detective named Robert Ledru. In 1887, Ledru was called to Le Havre to work on a case involving the disappearance of several seamen. After arriving and spending the night, he was reassigned: a man named André Monet had been found murdered on the beach. Ledru found footprints indicating the suspect had nine toes and a bullet that had been fired from a German pistol. Ledru had nine toes and a German pistol. He turned himself in. Not believing his story, the officers put him in a cell for the night with a loaded gun. Ledru shot at officers in his sleep. He spent the rest of his life under twenty-four-hour surveillance on a farm outside of Paris.

myth. In fact, it's more dangerous to leave them wandering around. It is, however, possible that they may lash out in confusion, inadvertently hurting whoever's doing the waking. It's best to gently lead them back to bed.

Sleepwalking rarely requires treatment. It's most common in young children and typically goes away of its own accord. For persistent sleepwalkers, treatments include improving sleep hygiene, hypnosis and the prescription of sedative drugs or antidepressants.

NIGHTMARE DISORDER

Most of us experience nightmares, whether they're quietly strange and unsettling or manic displays of gore and violence. They can be taut psychological thrillers or Tarantino movies. They can launch us from our beds and send us rocketing through our houses, flicking on every light switch and double-checking the lock on every window.

Unless times are particularly turbulent, though, they don't tend to happen too often. Not as often as they did when we were young, anyway. But for some people, nightmares are a constant plague that crop up almost every night and have cripplingly adverse effects on their lives. It's a formally recognized condition called nightmare disorder, categorized by the *Diagnostic and Statistical Manual of Mental Disorders* as:

A. Repeated awakenings from the major sleep period or naps with detailed recall of extended and extremely frightening dreams, usually involving threats to survival, security, or self-esteem. The awakenings generally occur during the second half of the sleep period.

B. On awakening from the frightening dreams, the person rapidly becomes oriented and alert (in contrast to the confusion and disorientation seen in sleep terror disorder and some forms of epilepsy).

C. The dream experience, or the sleep disturbance resulting from the awakening, causes clinically significant distress or impairment in social, occupational or other important areas of functioning.

Individuals suffering from nightmare disorder are likely to suffer from sleep deprivation, partly because they're afraid to fall asleep and partly because when they do manage to drift off, they're more likely to be woken by the terror of their dreams.

Nightmare disorder is often linked to mental health conditions, such as PTSD, borderline personality disorder and dissociative disorder, though it can also be caused by drug use, certain medications and a high-stress lifestyle. Treatment tends to involve a number of different strategies. Improved sleep hygiene, meditation and even lucid dreaming have all proven effective in combating persistent nightmares.

Unless you find them interfering with your daily life, nightmares shouldn't be a cause for concern – they're a natural, normal part of sleep and dreaming. Often bad dreams serve to draw our attention to issues that need dealing with, and go on to provide us with an arena in which we can practise dealing with them.

One study of former American soldiers showed that those who played video games typically experienced fewer nightmares, and the nightmares they did experience were of a decreased intensity. This is likely due to desensitization. However, when the study was repeated on women, the reverse was found to be true.

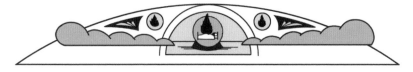

THE USES OF DREAMS

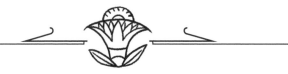

AN ANCIENT TOOL

'A dream! My sister, listen to my dream: Rushes are torn out for me; rushes keep growing for me. A single growing reed shakes its head for me. A twin reed, one is removed from me. Tall trees in the forest are uprooted by themselves for me. Water is poured over my pure hearth. The bottom of my pure churn drops away. My pure drinking cup is torn down from the peg where it hung. My shepherd's crook has disappeared from me. An eagle seizes a lamb from the sheepfold. A falcon catches a sparrow on the reed fence. My goats drag their lapis lazuli beards in the dust for me. My male sheep scratch the earth with thick legs for me. The churn lies on its side, no milk is poured. The cup lies on its side; Dumuzid lives no more. The sheepfold is given to the winds.'

The above text is a translation of the first ever recorded dream, written sometime around 3000 BCE by a Mesopotamian king named Dumuzid the Shepherd. At the time, huge significance was placed on dreams and they were often used as tools of political as well as personal guidance.

The interpretation of dreams was a task reserved for a special class of female priest, or 'questioner' as they were sometimes known. In a manner not dissimilar to this book, the dream priestess would ask the dreamer questions meant to flesh out and clarify the dream. Where did it take place? What role did you play? Which gods were present? The priestess would then go on to deconstruct any metaphors that could be identified in the tale, just as many dreamers attempt to do today, even consulting dream keys written on tablets.

We are told that Dumuzid's dream was interpreted for him by his sister, Geshtinanna. 'The rushes which keep growing thick about you are your demons,' she said, 'who will rise against you and ambush you.'

The Egyptians based their dream lore largely on that of the Mesopotamians. Again, dreams were considered predictions of the future, sent as messages from the gods, and were consulted for everything from where to build grain stores to how to cure illnesses.

 Egyptians were also pioneers of a form of lucid dreaming. It was widely believed that, if correctly harnessed, dreams could be used to explore alternative realities, pay a visit to the afterlife or spend time inside the minds of wild creatures.

It was believed that dreams regarding certain aspects of life had to be sent by the god in control of that aspect, and this was achieved by a practice known as 'incubation'. Egyptians would fast for several days, journey to a sleep temple built for the god they were seeking answers from, and perform a number of rites and prayers before falling asleep on a purpose-built bed. Once they'd received their dream, they'd likely go to a dream priest to have it interpreted.

The Egyptians had a number of their own dream books, the most notable dating back to the reign of Ramesses II (1279–1213 BCE). The book claimed that if a man sees himself drinking warm beer, it means suffering will follow. And if he sees himself killing a hippopotamus, it means a big meal is coming. While if a man sees himself caring for monkeys, it means change is on its way. Though these might not seem desperately relevant to us, they also wrote about the meaning of losing your teeth and of seeing yourself dead. It seems some stories are innate.

While the Greeks still relied on dreams as a means of divining the future, they were also the first to suggest they could be indicators of psychological or physical conditions. Hippocrates, often hailed as the father of modern medicine, thought that dreams, rather than being god-sent, came from within and were the body's way of communicating its problems. He claimed that if the world is dreamt as it is, and the events that take place in dreams are unremarkable, then the body is healthy. If, however, odd and fantastical dreams occur, then something is imbalanced or diseased, and the dream should be used as a means of diagnosis.

With these three ancient cultures, the foundations of modern dream interpretation had been laid. The history of humans and dreaming spans civilizations, and, while the importance placed on them may have shifted, our ways

'A dream which is not interpreted, is like a letter which is not read.' – the Talmud

and means of making sense of them remain strangely similar. Dreams remain one of the most ancient tools we use to navigate through our lives.

PROPHECIEſ ∧ND REVEL∧TIONſ

Since there have been dreams, there have been people hailing them as prophetic. From the ancient civilizations to the present day, people have long searched their dreams for clues of what tomorrow might bring.

The Bible is rife with night-time prophecy: from Micaiah's vision of the death of King Ahab, to Daniel's vision of the fall of Medo-Persia to Alexander the Great, and Joseph's dream of fleeing Egypt with Jesus to escape Herod's grasp. Often these experiences blur the line between prophecy and revelation. Sometimes they're presented more as survival tips sent from God, while other times they seem to be complex metaphors for how the proceeding centuries will play out.

Other well-known precognitive dreams tend to be framed in a supernatural context rather than a religious one: Abraham Lincoln supposedly spent three consecutive nights dreaming of his own funeral before he was assassinated while attending the theatre; there are at least ten corroborated accounts of people dreaming of the *Titanic* sinking; and the dreams of an Irish engineer called J.W. Dunne appeared to predict a volcanic eruption in the Caribbean, a factory fire in Paris, and the derailing of *The Flying Scotsman*.

Dunne went on to become one of the foremost proponents of the prophetic power of dreams. In a book titled *An Experiment with Time*, Dunne claimed that time was not linear, and that in a higher dimension, past, present, and future exist simultaneously. It was his belief that in dreams we're granted access to this dimension, thus enabling us to gain a glimpse of the future.

Dreams that appear to predict future events are mostly dismissed by scientists as the result either of memory bias or statistics. The former meaning that we're more likely to remember dreams which appear to foretell things in our lives, the latter meaning that on a planet of six billion people, a few are going to dream of the *Titanic* sinking the night before it actually does. Even Aristotle described precognitive dreams as 'mere coincidences'.

But this doesn't completely rule out dreams as useless predictors of tomorrow. For example, many women dream of being pregnant only to find out in the following weeks that in fact they are. This probably happens simply because in a dream state we're open to receiving information from the subconscious. On a more day-to-day basis, this might help us to better prepare for the future. For example, if you dream of doing badly in your driving test, it may be because some part of you is acknowledging that you're not yet ready or haven't had sufficient practice.

Although we're unlikely to be able to predict lottery numbers or volcanic eruptions, we might be able to predict certain things about ourselves. Perhaps not as prophecies, but at least as revelations from the subconscious.

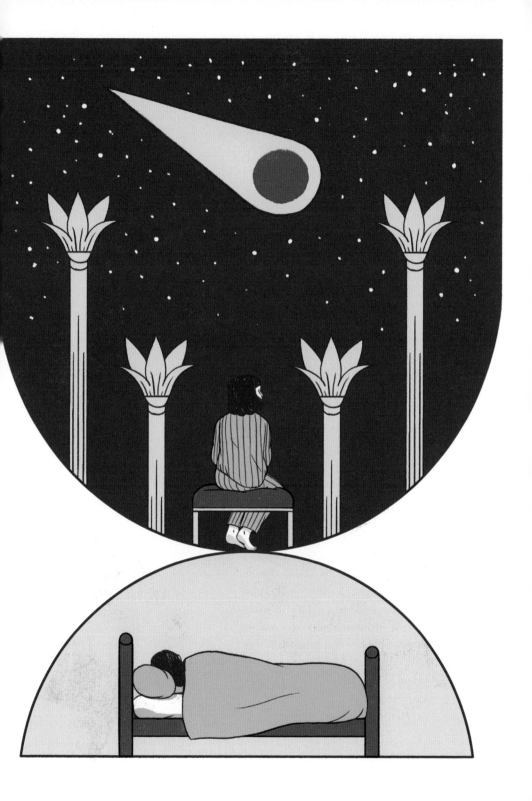

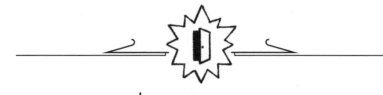

I**N**ſ**PIR**A**TION**

There are countless instances of artists, writers, scientists and people in all manner of professions that have reported gaining inspiration from dreams. Some seem to have come from nowhere, while others present themselves as solutions to problems that the dreamer has long been pondering. Without them, it's not hard to imagine that the world would be a very different place.

• In 1619, Descartes dreamt of being given a melon in a windstorm and woke inspired to create the scientific method still in use today.

• In 1797, Coleridge dreamt of thirteenth-century China after taking opium, and, after waking, immediately penned 'Kubla Khan', one of the most seminal Romantic poems.

• In 1816, somewhat disturbed by the tales of terror told by her holiday companions (Lord Byron, Percy Bysshe Shelley and John William Polidori), Mary Shelley had a dream about a terrible humanoid who was brought to life under the watchful eye of a young scientist. Some say this dream inspired her to write *Frankenstein; or, The Modern Prometheus*.

 Salvador Dalí utilized a method called 'slumber with a key' to find inspiration. It involves sitting with a heavy key over a metal pot and allowing yourself to drift into sleep. As soon as you get there, paralysis will take over and the key will fall, hitting the pot and waking you up. The benefit is the time spent in the hypnagogic state, which comes immediately before sleep and sees the brain at its most fluid and creative.

- In 1886, Robert Louis Stevenson dreamt of Dr Jekyll transforming into the monstrous Hyde and woke to write the entire novella in the space of three days.

- In 1905, Einstein dreamt of cows being electrocuted and woke to propose his theory of relativity.

- In 1913, Niels Bohr dreamt of electrons circling the nucleus of an atom like planets around a sun and was later awarded a Nobel Prize for the discovery.

- In 1953, Dr James Watson dreamt of intertwined serpents and woke to discover the double helix of DNA.

- In 1965, Paul McCartney dreamt of a melody he thought he'd heard in childhood, and woke to record 'Yesterday', which went on to become the most covered song in existence.

- In 1981, James Cameron dreamt of a chrome torso dragging itself along the floor with kitchen knives and woke to pen the script for *Terminator*, a franchise that has gone on to make almost two billion dollars at the box office.

- In 2003, Stephanie Meyer had one of the most important dreams of her life. 'I can still see it. It was a strange dream. I was looking at a circular meadow, in which a boy and a girl were talking. She was normal, but he sparkled in the sunshine. He was handsome. And he was a vampire.' When she woke, she wrote about her dream in one go and today that account is Chapter 13 of *Twilight*.

Whether or not you believe that dreams can be a link to supernatural worlds, or offer us messages from the gods, it's clear that they can provide artistic fuel, personal insight and new ways of looking at the world.

INSTRUCTION MANUAL TO
LEARN HOW TO DREAM

(and to know how to explain your dreams)

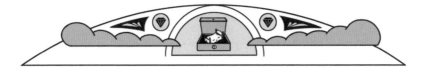

Holding on
to your dreams

Why keep a dream diary?

'Dreaming is an act of pure imagination, attesting in all men a creative power, which if it were available in waking, would make every man a Dante or Shakespeare.'
Francis Herbert Hedge

The biggest reason for keeping a dream diary is that if you don't, your dreams will be lost. Minutes and hours, totalling days and months, of your own worlds and creations will be irretrievably gone. By writing out your dreams, you'll transfer them into your long-term memory, and those incredible, vivid experiences you wake up with will sit waiting for you in the pages of this book, ready to be revisited like old photographs.

And why would you want to revisit your dreams? Hopefully the previous pages will have highlighted a few possibilities. Dreams can provide us with insights into ourselves, our psyches and our bodies. They can offer creative inspiration and solutions to stubborn problems. Dreams can allay anxieties, manage traumas and force us to confront our fears. They can also just be fun.

If your goal is lucid dreaming, keeping a diary will help to get you there. By cultivating self-awareness, you'll find yourself more able to engage reality checks, understand when you're dreaming, and ultimately end up on some unbelievable escapades. A dream diary can also have more immediate applications. If you wake up alone and startled after a particularly harrowing nightmare, writing it down and then altering the ending to something hilarious or absurd has been shown to help people calm down and get back to sleep. It goes back to the Boggarts and defeating shadows by laughing at them.

Keeping this dream diary can also be treated as a purely literary exercise. After all, dreams are stories, effortlessly spun and endlessly exciting. For a writer, having a book filled with imaginary creatures, characters and places will prove to be nothing short of a godsend.

So there are any number of reasons to keep a dream diary, and the best way of finding out what they are is to try it. Dreams help different people in different ways. You might be surprised by what you'll learn.

How to use this book

The key to getting the most from this book lies in integrating it into your daily routine. Once you get used to recording your dreams, not only will the act of writing them down get easier but the ease with which you remember them will improve too. The more you look, the more you'll see.

It's your book and it's yours to use how you want. Maybe you want to dive straight into the dream pages, maybe you want to plan things first in the Dreamcatcher section, which is at the back of this book. But here's our suggestion of how to get the most out of it:

1. On waking, immediately flick to the Dreamcatcher section and start scribbling down anything you can remember. Words, characters, feelings, whatever comes to mind. If it's easier to draw it, do that. Don't worry about spelling, grammar or even coherent sentences – all that matters is it being understandable to you.

2. Once you've got the basics of the dream down, you can start filling in a set of dream pages (you won't want to move past step one for every dream, just the ones that feel most special or potentially useful). For each dream, there are four pages. The first two pages deal with the specifics of date, place, content and emotion. The sooner this is done, the easier it will be, as the dream will still be fresh in your mind. If you don't have a lot of time, don't worry, just make sure your jottings have as much in them as possible.

3. Give your dream a title, something that will help you to remember it. If the dream was lucid, put an asterisk by its name so you can tally them up.

4. Write out the story of your dream. This can be in whatever form you want, with as much detail as you feel is necessary. A poem, a story, song lyrics. Whatever you feel will help you to remember.

5. The next section is for drawing conclusions from your dream. What can you do with this? Why did you dream this? What could the symbols mean? This book has purposely avoided including any real kind of dream key. You'll be far better at deciphering your own metaphors than we could ever be.

6. After cataloguing a number of your dreams, you may find it useful to go back and look for any recurring themes, symbols or correlations. Did certain kinds of dreams happen in certain places? Or after seeing certain people? After eating certain types of cheese?

It doesn't matter if you don't write every week, or even every month. It doesn't matter if you leave most of your dreams as notes in the Dreamcatcher section or doodles in the margins of these chapters. It doesn't even matter if you only use the following pages once. If this book can save any of your dreams from disappearing into the abyss, it will have been worthwhile. Good luck and goodnight.

A PRACTICAL EXAMPLE

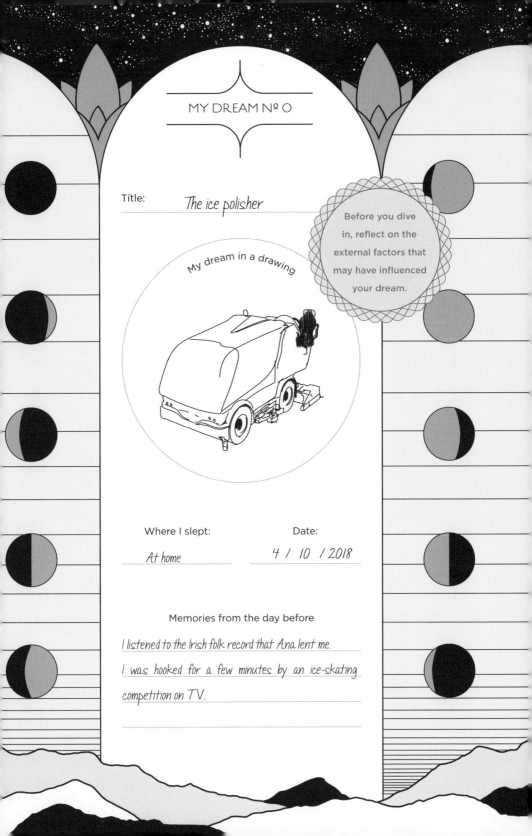

MY DREAM № 0

Title: *The ice polisher*

My dream in a drawing

Before you dive in, reflect on the external factors that may have influenced your dream.

Where I slept:

At home

Date:

4 / 10 / 2018

Memories from the day before

I listened to the Irish folk record that Ana lent me.

I was hooked for a few minutes by an ice-skating

competition on TV.

DECONSTRUCTING MY DREAM

My role in the dream: *I'm in charge of the ice polisher used on a skating rink in the centre of Dublin.*

These details will help you to deconstruct your dream. They are essential for you to work out what your dream is trying to tell you.

(●) Protagonist   ( ) Secondary role   ( ) Not present

Other characters:
_____

Feelings:

Stress

Enthusiasm

Locations / places:

Dublin

Local ice-skating rink

Objects:

My mobile phone and earphones

Sounds:

Squeaks when polishing the ice

Irish folk music

Genre:

( ) Nightmare
( ) Fantasy
(●) Symbolic
( ) Everyday
( ) Surreal
( ) Erotic

Place in time:

( ) A while ago
( ) Recent past
( ) Present day
(●) Near future
( ) Distant future
( ) Unknown

Type:

( ) Lucid
( ) Recurring
(●) Unfinished
( ) False awakening
( ) Episodic
( ) Blurry

THE STORY OF MY DREAM

In a fit of madness, I decide to leave my home and move to Dublin, where I work at a giant ice-skating rink at night-time. I have been employed only for a short while, so I'm not very good with the polisher and I'm a little anxious that I'll get things wrong.

It turns out I'm right to be worried, because a hole in the ice appears a few metres away. I worry that I'll create lots of holes in the ice, so I decide to play music to relax. I play the record I've been listening to on a loop for months.

Surprisingly, the polisher seems more manageable with the background music, and I even feel happy enough to start singing along to a couple of songs. I don't mess up even when I'm driving with one hand and singing into an invisible microphone.

When I put the polisher back, I look at the rink and see that it is perfect.

This is the page where you will take your time and write about your dream in full. There are pages at the end of the diary called Dreamcatcher, where you can write down hurried ideas.

CONCLUSIONS

Why I had this dream and how it can be useful to me

I think I should start listening to more varied music, because my obsession with Irish folk is starting to dominate everything. As in my dream, I've just started a new job and I'm worried about not getting through my probation period. Each hole in the ice may be an email that I don't know how to answer. It also explains the sudden perfectionism that lately I'm barely able to control and is driving my flatmates mad. My decision to listen to music to relax probably means that I can do it by approaching things more calmly. The reason my shift on the rink is at night is because I'm not good at switching off and relaxing.

Reread your dream calmly. Try, on the one hand, to analyse what's in your life that led you to your dream. Then think about how can you apply all that you have learnt from writing about your dream to your life.

— END OF THE DREAM —

WELCOME TO THE DIARY
OF YOUR DREAMS

This is where you record, develop and narrate your dreams
(as well as learn from them)

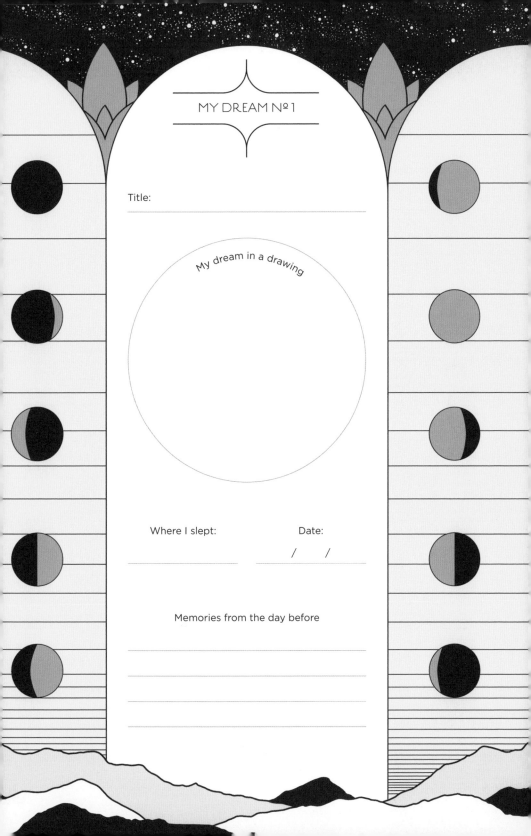

MY DREAM №1

Title:
_____

My dream in a drawing

Where I slept: Date:

_____   ___ / ___ / ___

Memories from the day before

_____
_____
_____
_____

DECONSTRUCTING MY DREAM

My role in the dream:

_____

_____

_____

◯ Protagonist   ◯ Secondary role   ◯ Not present

Other characters:

_____

_____

Feelings:

_____

_____

_____

_____

Locations / places:

_____

_____

_____

_____

Objects:

_____

_____

Sounds:

_____

_____

Genre:

◯ Nightmare
◯ Fantasy
◯ Symbolic
◯ Everyday
◯ Surreal
◯ Erotic

Place in time:

◯ A while ago
◯ Recent past
◯ Present day
◯ Near future
◯ Distant future
◯ Unknown

Type:

◯ Lucid
◯ Recurring
◯ Unfinished
◯ False awakening
◯ Episodic
◯ Blurry

THE STORY OF MY DREAM

CONCLUSIONS

Why I had this dream and how it can be useful to me

_____

_____

_____

_____

_____

_____

_____

_____

_____

_____

_____

_____

_____

_____

_____

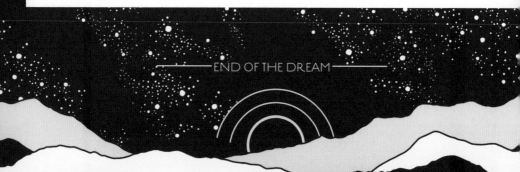

END OF THE DREAM

MY DREAM № 2

Title:

My dream in a drawing

Where I slept: Date:

/   /

Memories from the day before

DECONSTRUCTING MY DREAM

My role in the dream:

_____

_____

_____

( ) Protagonist   ( ) Secondary role   ( ) Not present

Other characters:

_____

_____

Feelings:

_____

_____

_____

_____

Locations / places:

_____

_____

_____

_____

Objects:

_____

_____

Sounds:

_____

_____

Genre:

( ) Nightmare
( ) Fantasy
( ) Symbolic
( ) Everyday
( ) Surreal
( ) Erotic

Place in time:

( ) A while ago
( ) Recent past
( ) Present day
( ) Near future
( ) Distant future
( ) Unknown

Type:

( ) Lucid
( ) Recurring
( ) Unfinished
( ) False awakening
( ) Episodic
( ) Blurry

THE STORY OF MY DREAM

CONCLUSIONS

Why I had this dream and how it can be useful to me

_____

_____

_____

_____

_____

_____

_____

_____

_____

_____

_____

_____

_____

_____

_____

_____

END OF THE DREAM

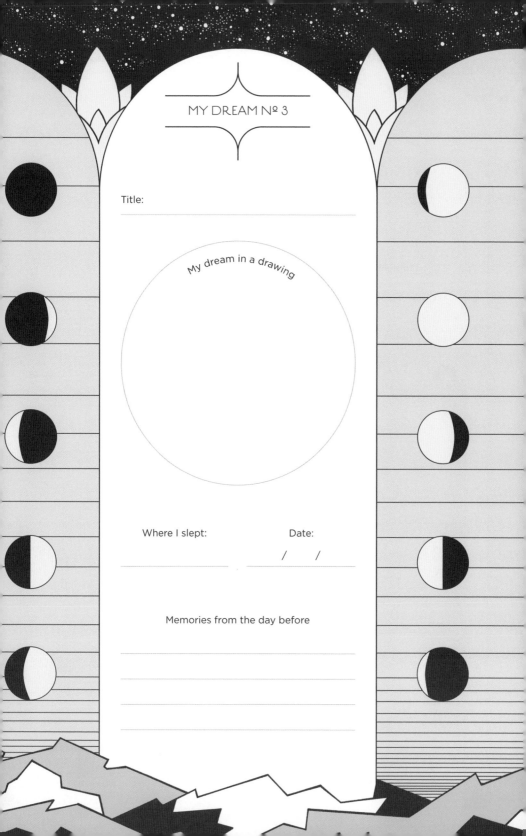

MY DREAM № 3

Title:

My dream in a drawing

Where I slept: Date:
                                    /   /

Memories from the day before

DECONSTRUCTING MY DREAM

My role in the dream:

_____

_____

_____

◯ Protagonist ◯ Secondary role ◯ Not present

Other characters:

_____

_____

Feelings:

_____

_____

_____

_____

Locations / places:

_____

_____

_____

_____

Objects:

_____

_____

Sounds:

_____

_____

Genre:

◯ Nightmare
◯ Fantasy
◯ Symbolic
◯ Everyday
◯ Surreal
◯ Erotic

Place in time:

◯ A while ago
◯ Recent past
◯ Present day
◯ Near future
◯ Distant future
◯ Unknown

Type:

◯ Lucid
◯ Recurring
◯ Unfinished
◯ False awakening
◯ Episodic
◯ Blurry

THE STORY OF MY DREAM

CONCLUSIONS

Why I had this dream and how it can be useful to me

_____

_____

_____

_____

_____

_____

_____

_____

_____

_____

_____

_____

_____

_____

_____

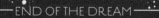 END OF THE DREAM

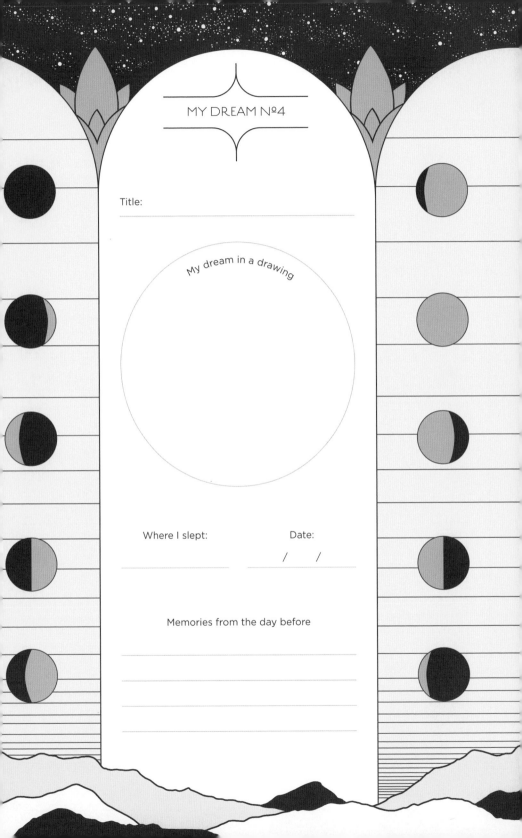

MY DREAM Nº4

Title:
_____

My dream in a drawing

Where I slept: Date:

_____   ___/___/___

Memories from the day before

_____
_____
_____
_____

DECONSTRUCTING MY DREAM

My role in the dream:

_____

_____

_____

◯ Protagonist   ◯ Secondary role   ◯ Not present

Other characters:

_____

_____

Feelings:

_____

_____

_____

_____

Locations / places:

_____

_____

_____

_____

Objects:

_____

_____

Sounds:

_____

_____

Genre:
◯ Nightmare
◯ Fantasy
◯ Symbolic
◯ Everyday
◯ Surreal
◯ Erotic

Place in time:
◯ A while ago
◯ Recent past
◯ Present day
◯ Near future
◯ Distant future
◯ Unknown

Type:
◯ Lucid
◯ Recurring
◯ Unfinished
◯ False awakening
◯ Episodic
◯ Blurry

THE STORY OF MY DREAM

CONCLUSIONS

Why I had this dream and how it can be useful to me

_____

_____

_____

_____

_____

_____

_____

_____

_____

_____

_____

_____

_____

_____

_____

——— END OF THE DREAM ———

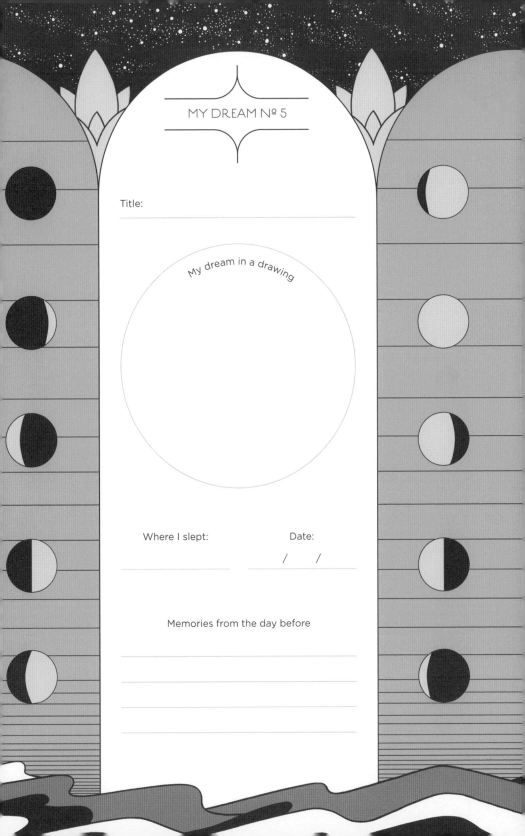

MY DREAM № 5

Title:
_____

My dream in a drawing

Where I slept: Date:
_____   ___ / ___ / ___

Memories from the day before

_____
_____
_____
_____

DECONSTRUCTING MY DREAM

My role in the dream:

_____

_____

_____

◯ Protagonist　　◯ Secondary role　　◯ Not present

Other characters:

_____

_____

Feelings:

_____

_____

_____

_____

Locations / places:

_____

_____

_____

_____

Objects:

_____

_____

Sounds:

_____

_____

Genre:

◯ Nightmare
◯ Fantasy
◯ Symbolic
◯ Everyday
◯ Surreal
◯ Erotic

Place in time:

◯ A while ago
◯ Recent past
◯ Present day
◯ Near future
◯ Distant future
◯ Unknown

Type:

◯ Lucid
◯ Recurring
◯ Unfinished
◯ False awakening
◯ Episodic
◯ Blurry

THE STORY OF MY DREAM

CONCLUSIONS

Why I had this dream and how it can be useful to me

_____

_____

_____

_____

_____

_____

_____

_____

_____

_____

_____

_____

_____

_____

_____

_____

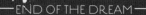 END OF THE DREAM

MY DREAM № 6

Title:
_____

My dream in a drawing

Where I slept: Date:

_____   ___/___/___

Memories from the day before

_____
_____
_____

DECONSTRUCTING MY DREAM

My role in the dream:

_____

_____

_____

◯ Protagonist   ◯ Secondary role   ◯ Not present

Other characters:

_____

_____

Feelings:

_____

_____

_____

_____

Locations / places:

_____

_____

_____

_____

Objects:

_____

_____

Sounds:

_____

_____

Genre:

◯ Nightmare
◯ Fantasy
◯ Symbolic
◯ Everyday
◯ Surreal
◯ Erotic

Place in time:

◯ A while ago
◯ Recent past
◯ Present day
◯ Near future
◯ Distant future
◯ Unknown

Type:

◯ Lucid
◯ Recurring
◯ Unfinished
◯ False awakening
◯ Episodic
◯ Blurry

THE STORY OF MY DREAM

CONCLUSIONS

Why I had this dream and how it can be useful to me

_____

_____

_____

_____

_____

_____

_____

_____

_____

_____

_____

_____

_____

_____

_____

_____

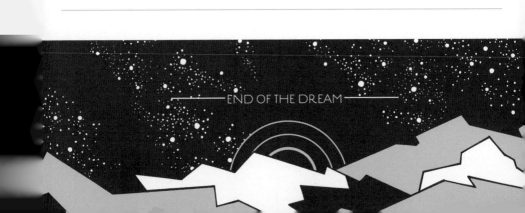

END OF THE DREAM

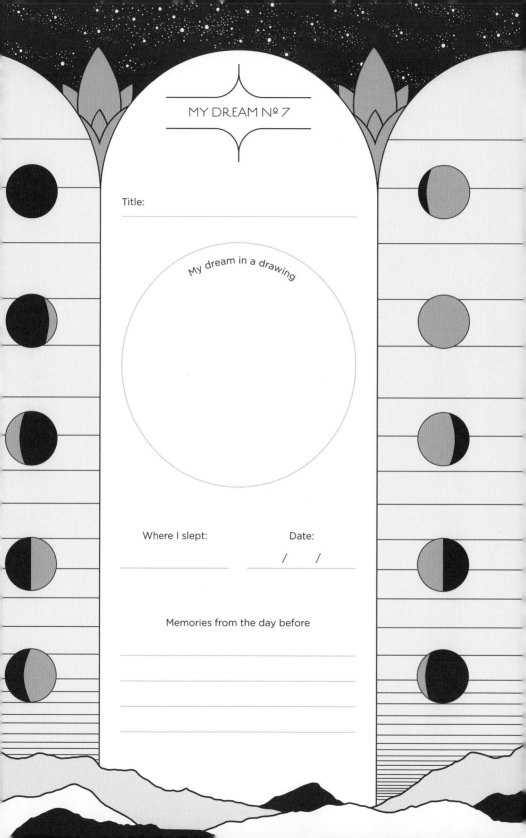

MY DREAM Nº 7

Title:

My dream in a drawing

Where I slept:

Date:
/   /

Memories from the day before

DECONSTRUCTING MY DREAM

My role in the dream:

_____

_____

_____

◯ Protagonist   ◯ Secondary role   ◯ Not present

Other characters:

_____

_____

Feelings:

_____

_____

_____

Locations / places:

_____

_____

_____

Objects:

_____

_____

Sounds:

_____

_____

Genre:

◯ Nightmare
◯ Fantasy
◯ Symbolic
◯ Everyday
◯ Surreal
◯ Erotic

Place in time:

◯ A while ago
◯ Recent past
◯ Present day
◯ Near future
◯ Distant future
◯ Unknown

Type:

◯ Lucid
◯ Recurring
◯ Unfinished
◯ False awakening
◯ Episodic
◯ Blurry

THE STORY OF MY DREAM

CONCLUSIONS

Why I had this dream and how it can be useful to me

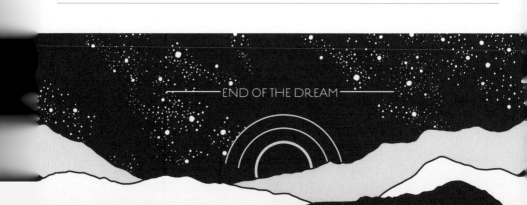

END OF THE DREAM

MY DREAM № 8

Title:

My dream in a drawing

Where I slept:

Date:

/　　/

Memories from the day before

DECONSTRUCTING MY DREAM

My role in the dream:

_____

_____

_____

◯ Protagonist   ◯ Secondary role   ◯ Not present

Other characters:

_____

_____

Feelings:

_____

_____

_____

_____

Locations / places:

_____

_____

_____

_____

Objects:

_____

_____

_____

Sounds:

_____

_____

_____

Genre:

◯ Nightmare
◯ Fantasy
◯ Symbolic
◯ Everyday
◯ Surreal
◯ Erotic

Place in time:

◯ A while ago
◯ Recent past
◯ Present day
◯ Near future
◯ Distant future
◯ Unknown

Type:

◯ Lucid
◯ Recurring
◯ Unfinished
◯ False awakening
◯ Episodic
◯ Blurry

THE STORY OF MY DREAM

CONCLUSIONS

Why I had this dream and how it can be useful to me

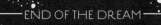

END OF THE DREAM

MY DREAM № 9

Title:

_____

My dream in a drawing

Where I slept: Date:

_____   ___ / ___ / ___

Memories from the day before

....

....

....

....

DECONSTRUCTING MY DREAM

My role in the dream:

_____

_____

_____

◯ Protagonist   ◯ Secondary role   ◯ Not present

Other characters:

_____

_____

Feelings:

_____

_____

_____

_____

Locations / places:

_____

_____

_____

_____

Objects:

_____

_____

Sounds:

_____

_____

Genre:

◯ Nightmare
◯ Fantasy
◯ Symbolic
◯ Everyday
◯ Surreal
◯ Erotic

Place in time:

◯ A while ago
◯ Recent past
◯ Present day
◯ Near future
◯ Distant future
◯ Unknown

Type:

◯ Lucid
◯ Recurring
◯ Unfinished
◯ False awakening
◯ Episodic
◯ Blurry

THE STORY OF MY DREAM

CONCLUSIONS

Why I had this dream and how it can be useful to me

_____

_____

_____

_____

_____

_____

_____

_____

_____

_____

_____

_____

_____

_____

_____

_____

_____

——————— END OF THE DREAM ———————

MY DREAM № 10

Title:

My dream in a drawing

Where I slept:

Date:
/   /

Memories from the day before

DECONSTRUCTING MY DREAM

My role in the dream:

_____

_____

_____

◯ Protagonist ◯ Secondary role ◯ Not present

Other characters:

_____

_____

Feelings:

_____

_____

_____

_____

Locations / places:

_____

_____

_____

_____

Objects:

_____

_____

Sounds:

_____

_____

Genre:

◯ Nightmare
◯ Fantasy
◯ Symbolic
◯ Everyday
◯ Surreal
◯ Erotic

Place in time:

◯ A while ago
◯ Recent past
◯ Present day
◯ Near future
◯ Distant future
◯ Unknown

Type:

◯ Lucid
◯ Recurring
◯ Unfinished
◯ False awakening
◯ Episodic
◯ Blurry

THE STORY OF MY DREAM

CONCLUSIONS

Why I had this dream and how it can be useful to me

_____

_____

_____

_____

_____

_____

_____

_____

_____

_____

_____

_____

_____

_____

_____

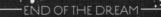

END OF THE DREAM

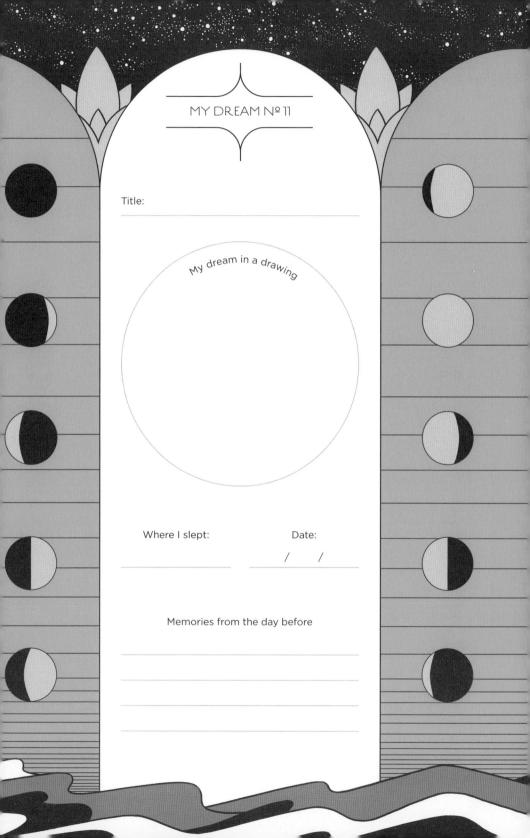

MY DREAM № 11

Title:
_____

My dream in a drawing

Where I slept: Date:
_____   ___ / ___ / ___

Memories from the day before

_____
_____
_____
_____

DECONSTRUCTING MY DREAM

My role in the dream:

_____

_____

_____

○ Protagonist   ○ Secondary role   ○ Not present

Other characters:

_____

_____

Feelings:

_____

_____

_____

_____

Locations / places:

_____

_____

_____

_____

Objects:

_____

_____

Sounds:

_____

_____

Genre:

○ Nightmare
○ Fantasy
○ Symbolic
○ Everyday
○ Surreal
○ Erotic

Place in time:

○ A while ago
○ Recent past
○ Present day
○ Near future
○ Distant future
○ Unknown

Type:

○ Lucid
○ Recurring
○ Unfinished
○ False awakening
○ Episodic
○ Blurry

THE STORY OF MY DREAM

CONCLUSIONS

Why I had this dream and how it can be useful to me

_____

_____

_____

_____

_____

_____

_____

_____

_____

_____

_____

_____

_____

_____

_____

_____

_____

_____

_____

————— END OF THE DREAM —————

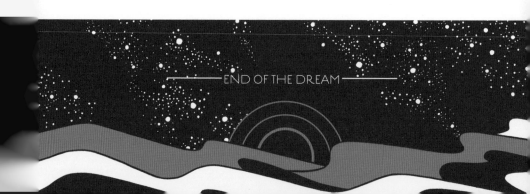

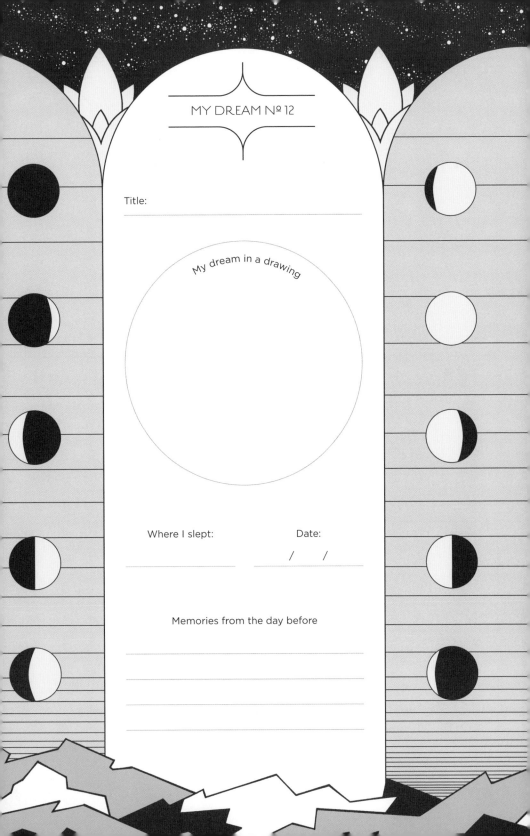

MY DREAM № 12

Title:

My dream in a drawing

Where I slept:

Date:

/   /

Memories from the day before

DECONSTRUCTING MY DREAM

My role in the dream:

_____

_____

_____

◯ Protagonist   ◯ Secondary role   ◯ Not present

Other characters:

_____

_____

Feelings:

_____

_____

_____

_____

Locations / places:

_____

_____

_____

_____

Objects:

_____

_____

Sounds:

_____

_____

Genre:

◯ Nightmare
◯ Fantasy
◯ Symbolic
◯ Everyday
◯ Surreal
◯ Erotic

Place in time:

◯ A while ago
◯ Recent past
◯ Present day
◯ Near future
◯ Distant future
◯ Unknown

Type:

◯ Lucid
◯ Recurring
◯ Unfinished
◯ False awakening
◯ Episodic
◯ Blurry

THE STORY OF MY DREAM

CONCLUSIONS

Why I had this dream and how it can be useful to me

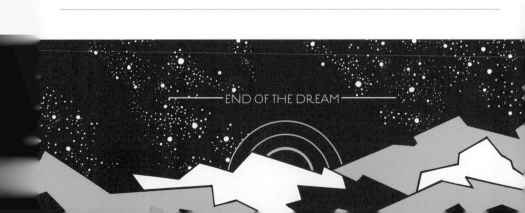

END OF THE DREAM

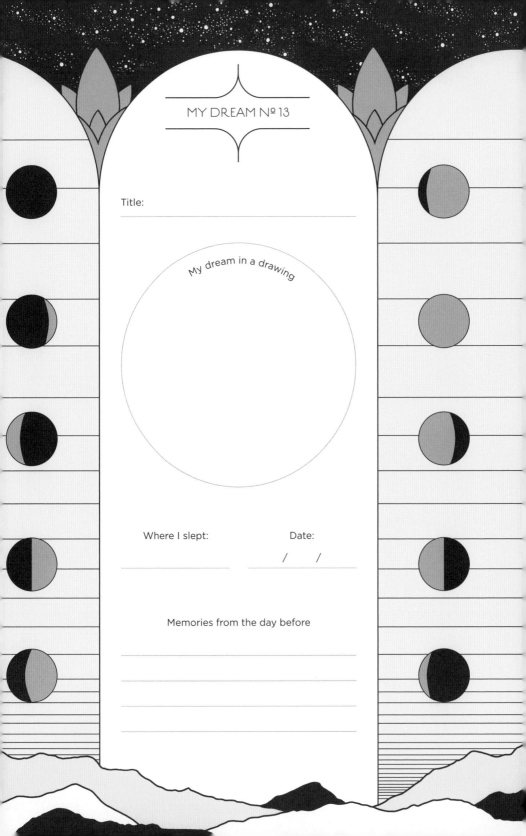

MY DREAM № 13

Title:
_____

My dream in a drawing

Where I slept: Date:
                            /   /
_____   _____

Memories from the day before
_____
_____
_____
_____

DECONSTRUCTING MY DREAM

My role in the dream:

_____

_____

_____

◯ Protagonist   ◯ Secondary role   ◯ Not present

Other characters:

_____

_____

Feelings:

_____

_____

_____

Locations / places:

_____

_____

_____

Objects:

_____

_____

Sounds:

_____

_____

Genre:

◯ Nightmare
◯ Fantasy
◯ Symbolic
◯ Everyday
◯ Surreal
◯ Erotic

Place in time:

◯ A while ago
◯ Recent past
◯ Present day
◯ Near future
◯ Distant future
◯ Unknown

Type:

◯ Lucid
◯ Recurring
◯ Unfinished
◯ False awakening
◯ Episodic
◯ Blurry

THE STORY OF MY DREAM

CONCLUSIONS

Why I had this dream and how it can be useful to me

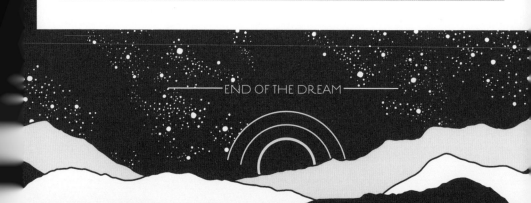

END OF THE DREAM

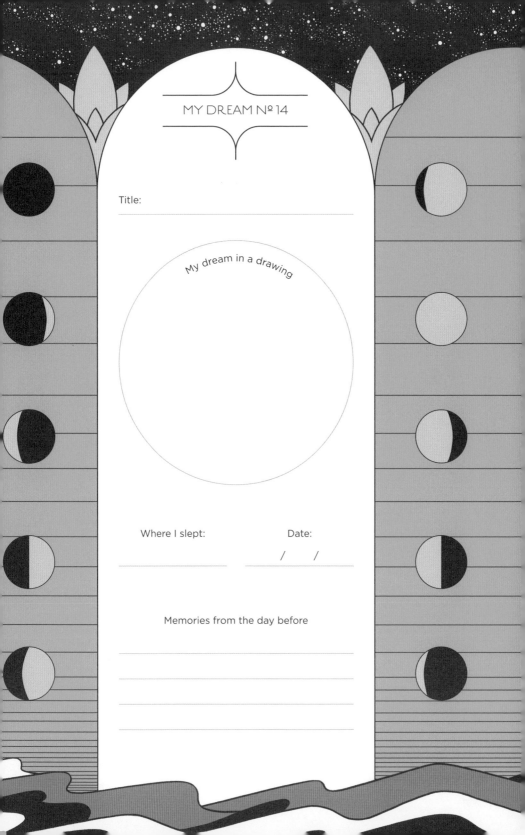

MY DREAM № 14

Title:

My dream in a drawing

Where I slept:

Date:

/   /

Memories from the day before

DECONSTRUCTING MY DREAM

My role in the dream:

_____

_____

_____

◯ Protagonist   ◯ Secondary role   ◯ Not present

Other characters:

_____

_____

Feelings:

_____

_____

_____

_____

Locations / places:

_____

_____

_____

_____

Objects:

_____

_____

_____

Sounds:

_____

_____

_____

Genre:

◯ Nightmare
◯ Fantasy
◯ Symbolic
◯ Everyday
◯ Surreal
◯ Erotic

Place in time:

◯ A while ago
◯ Recent past
◯ Present day
◯ Near future
◯ Distant future
◯ Unknown

Type:

◯ Lucid
◯ Recurring
◯ Unfinished
◯ False awakening
◯ Episodic
◯ Blurry

THE STORY OF MY DREAM

CONCLUSIONS

Why I had this dream and how it can be useful to me

_____

_____

_____

_____

_____

_____

_____

_____

_____

_____

_____

_____

_____

_____

_____

_____

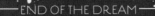

END OF THE DREAM

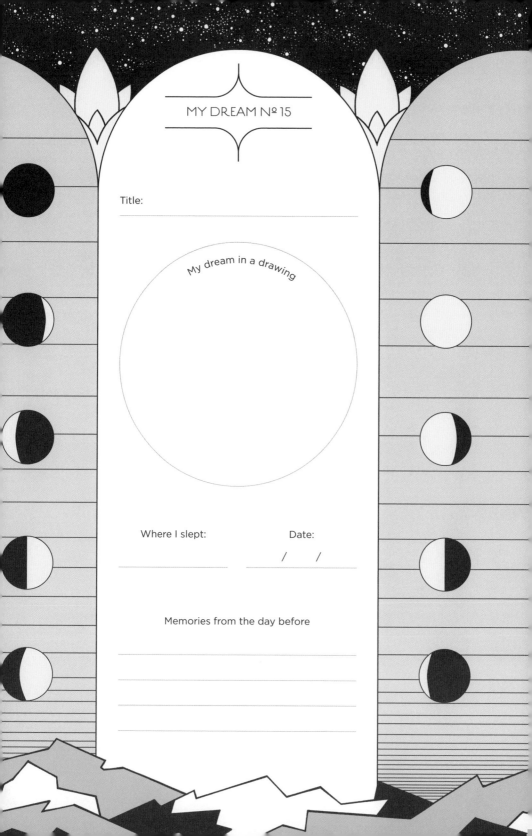

MY DREAM № 15

Title:

My dream in a drawing

Where I slept:

Date:

/   /

Memories from the day before

DECONSTRUCTING MY DREAM

My role in the dream:
_____
_____
_____

◯ Protagonist   ◯ Secondary role   ◯ Not present

Other characters:
_____
_____

Feelings:
_____
_____
_____
_____

Locations / places:
_____
_____
_____
_____

Objects:
_____
_____

Sounds:
_____
_____

Genre:
◯ Nightmare
◯ Fantasy
◯ Symbolic
◯ Everyday
◯ Surreal
◯ Erotic

Place in time:
◯ A while ago
◯ Recent past
◯ Present day
◯ Near future
◯ Distant future
◯ Unknown

Type:
◯ Lucid
◯ Recurring
◯ Unfinished
◯ False awakening
◯ Episodic
◯ Blurry

THE STORY OF MY DREAM

CONCLUSIONS

Why I had this dream and how it can be useful to me

_____

_____

_____

_____

_____

_____

_____

_____

_____

_____

_____

_____

_____

_____

_____

_____

_____

———————— END OF THE DREAM ————————

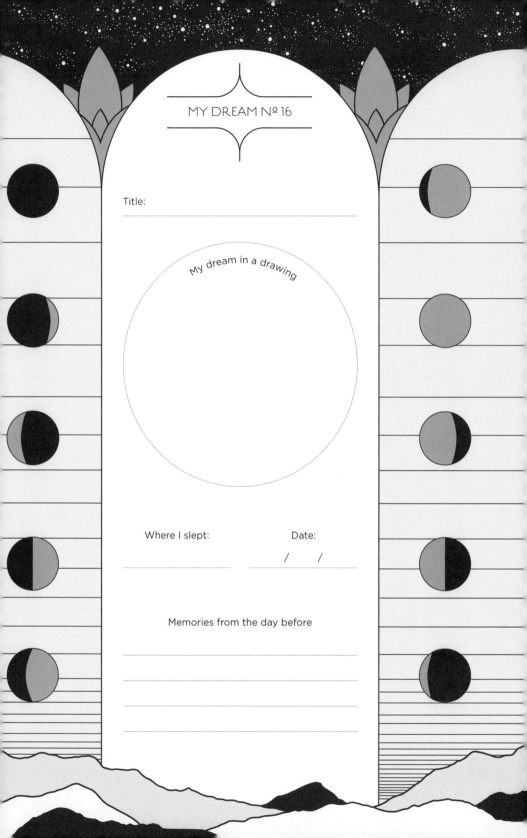

MY DREAM Nº 16

Title:
....

My dream in a drawing

Where I slept: Date:

_____   /   /

Memories from the day before

_____
_____
_____
_____

DECONSTRUCTING MY DREAM

My role in the dream:

_____

_____

_____

◯ Protagonist   ◯ Secondary role   ◯ Not present

Other characters:

_____

_____

Feelings:

_____

_____

_____

_____

Locations / places:

_____

_____

_____

_____

Objects:

_____

_____

Sounds:

_____

_____

Genre:

◯ Nightmare
◯ Fantasy
◯ Symbolic
◯ Everyday
◯ Surreal
◯ Erotic

Place in time:

◯ A while ago
◯ Recent past
◯ Present day
◯ Near future
◯ Distant future
◯ Unknown

Type:

◯ Lucid
◯ Recurring
◯ Unfinished
◯ False awakening
◯ Episodic
◯ Blurry

THE STORY OF MY DREAM

CONCLUSIONS

Why I had this dream and how it can be useful to me

_____

_____

_____

_____

_____

_____

_____

_____

_____

_____

_____

_____

_____

_____

_____

_____

————— END OF THE DREAM —————

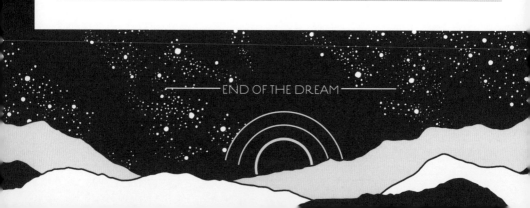

MY DREAM № 17

Title:
_____

My dream in a drawing

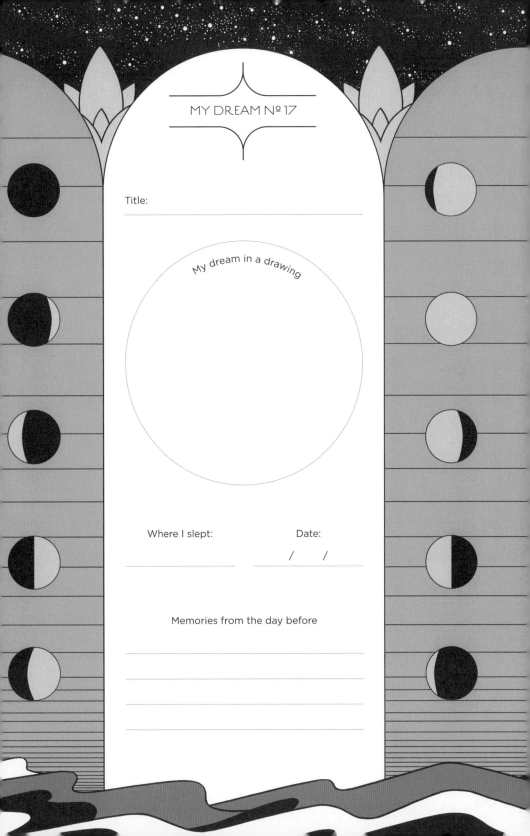

Where I slept: Date:

_____   _____
                                  /   /

Memories from the day before

_____
_____
_____
_____

DECONSTRUCTING MY DREAM

My role in the dream:

_____

_____

_____

◯ Protagonist   ◯ Secondary role   ◯ Not present

Other characters:

_____

_____

Feelings:

_____

_____

_____

Locations / places:

_____

_____

_____

Objects:

_____

_____

Sounds:

_____

_____

Genre:

◯ Nightmare
◯ Fantasy
◯ Symbolic
◯ Everyday
◯ Surreal
◯ Erotic

Place in time:

◯ A while ago
◯ Recent past
◯ Present day
◯ Near future
◯ Distant future
◯ Unknown

Type:

◯ Lucid
◯ Recurring
◯ Unfinished
◯ False awakening
◯ Episodic
◯ Blurry

THE STORY OF MY DREAM

CONCLUSIONS

Why I had this dream and how it can be useful to me

_____

_____

_____

_____

_____

_____

_____

_____

_____

_____

_____

_____

_____

_____

_____

_____

_____

END OF THE DREAM

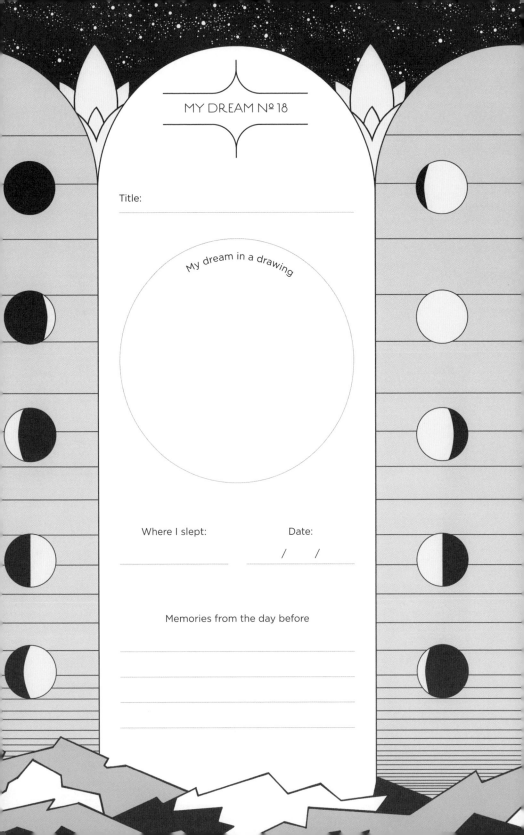

MY DREAM № 18

Title:

My dream in a drawing

Where I slept: Date:
                                   /   /

Memories from the day before

DECONSTRUCTING MY DREAM

My role in the dream:

_____

_____

_____

◯ Protagonist ◯ Secondary role ◯ Not present

Other characters:

_____

_____

Feelings:

_____

_____

_____

_____

Locations / places:

_____

_____

_____

_____

Objects:

_____

_____

Sounds:

_____

_____

Genre:

◯ Nightmare
◯ Fantasy
◯ Symbolic
◯ Everyday
◯ Surreal
◯ Erotic

Place in time:

◯ A while ago
◯ Recent past
◯ Present day
◯ Near future
◯ Distant future
◯ Unknown

Type:

◯ Lucid
◯ Recurring
◯ Unfinished
◯ False awakening
◯ Episodic
◯ Blurry

THE STORY OF MY DREAM

CONCLUSIONS

Why I had this dream and how it can be useful to me

_____

_____

_____

_____

_____

_____

_____

_____

_____

_____

_____

_____

_____

_____

_____

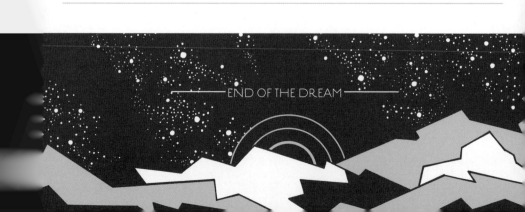

END OF THE DREAM

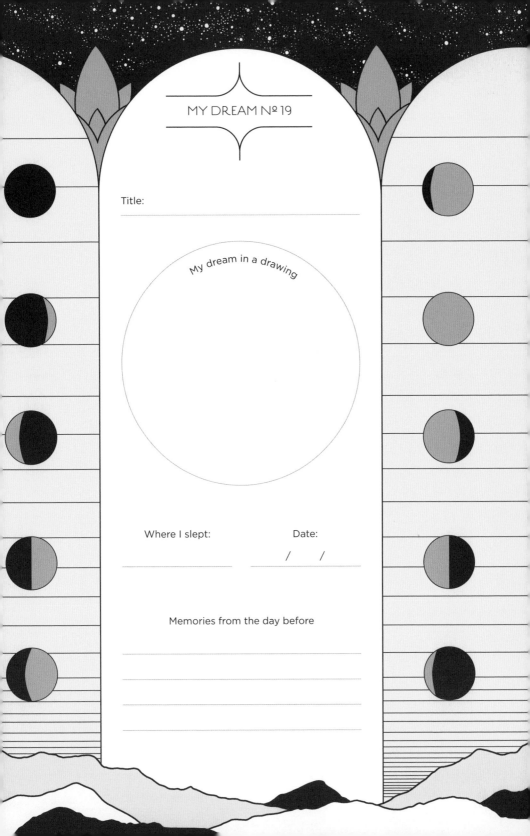

MY DREAM № 19

Title:

My dream in a drawing

Where I slept: Date:

                                   /   /

Memories from the day before

DECONSTRUCTING MY DREAM

My role in the dream:

_____

_____

_____

◯ Protagonist   ◯ Secondary role   ◯ Not present

Other characters:

_____

_____

Feelings:

_____

_____

_____

_____

Locations / places:

_____

_____

_____

_____

Objects:

_____

_____

Sounds:

_____

_____

Genre:

◯ Nightmare
◯ Fantasy
◯ Symbolic
◯ Everyday
◯ Surreal
◯ Erotic

Place in time:

◯ A while ago
◯ Recent past
◯ Present day
◯ Near future
◯ Distant future
◯ Unknown

Type:

◯ Lucid
◯ Recurring
◯ Unfinished
◯ False awakening
◯ Episodic
◯ Blurry

THE STORY OF MY DREAM

CONCLUSIONS

Why I had this dream and how it can be useful to me

_____

_____

_____

_____

_____

_____

_____

_____

_____

_____

_____

_____

_____

_____

_____

_____

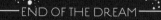

END OF THE DREAM

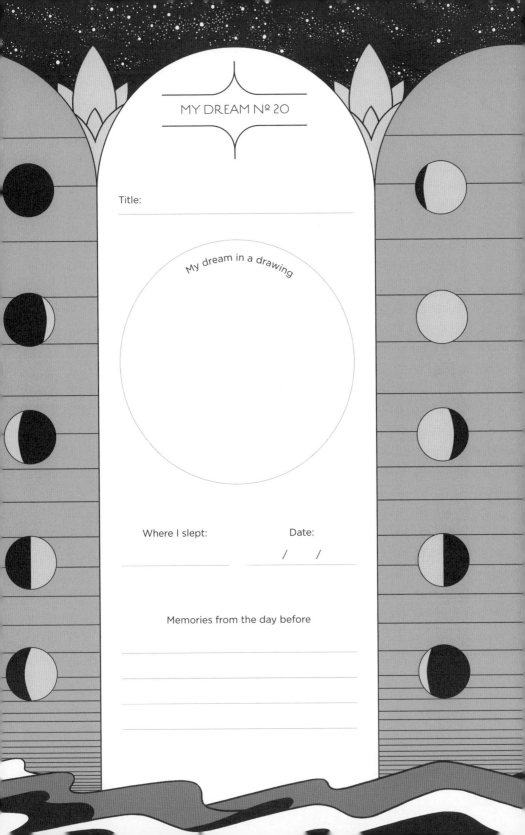

MY DREAM № 20

Title:
_____

My dream in a drawing

Where I slept: Date:

_____   /   /

Memories from the day before

_____
_____
_____
_____

DECONSTRUCTING MY DREAM

My role in the dream:

_____

_____

_____

◯ Protagonist   ◯ Secondary role   ◯ Not present

Other characters:

_____

_____

Feelings:	Locations / places:
_____	_____
_____	_____
_____	_____
_____	_____

Objects:	Sounds:
_____	_____
_____	_____

Genre:
◯ Nightmare
◯ Fantasy
◯ Symbolic
◯ Everyday
◯ Surreal
◯ Erotic

Place in time:
◯ A while ago
◯ Recent past
◯ Present day
◯ Near future
◯ Distant future
◯ Unknown

Type:
◯ Lucid
◯ Recurring
◯ Unfinished
◯ False awakening
◯ Episodic
◯ Blurry

THE STORY OF MY DREAM

CONCLUSIONS

Why I had this dream and how it can be useful to me

_____

_____

_____

_____

_____

_____

_____

_____

_____

_____

_____

_____

_____

_____

_____

_____

_____

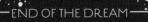

END OF THE DREAM

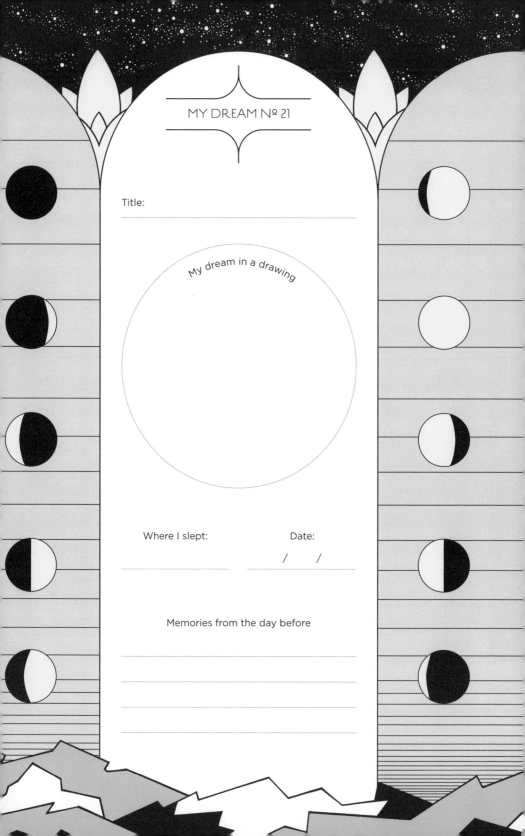

MY DREAM № 21

Title:
_____

My dream in a drawing

Where I slept: Date:
_____   /   /
_____

Memories from the day before

_____
_____
_____
_____

DECONSTRUCTING MY DREAM

My role in the dream:

_____

_____

_____

◯ Protagonist   ◯ Secondary role   ◯ Not present

Other characters:

_____

_____

Feelings:

_____

_____

_____

_____

Locations / places:

_____

_____

_____

_____

Objects:

_____

_____

Sounds:

_____

_____

Genre:

◯ Nightmare
◯ Fantasy
◯ Symbolic
◯ Everyday
◯ Surreal
◯ Erotic

Place in time:

◯ A while ago
◯ Recent past
◯ Present day
◯ Near future
◯ Distant future
◯ Unknown

Type:

◯ Lucid
◯ Recurring
◯ Unfinished
◯ False awakening
◯ Episodic
◯ Blurry

THE STORY OF MY DREAM

CONCLUSIONS

Why I had this dream and how it can be useful to me

_____
_____
_____
_____
_____
_____
_____
_____
_____
_____
_____
_____
_____

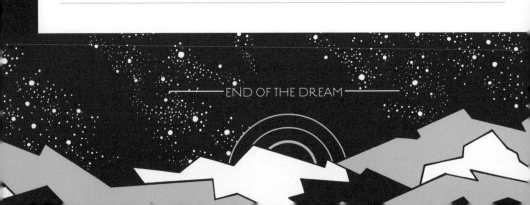

END OF THE DREAM

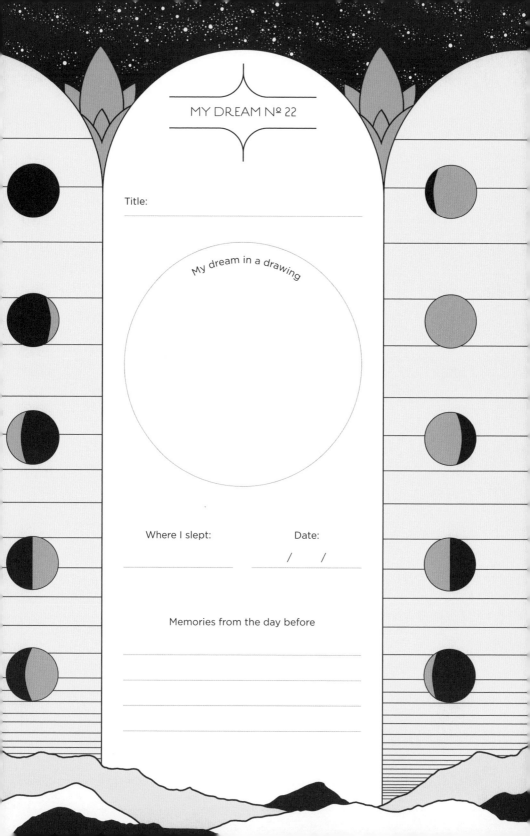

MY DREAM № 22

Title:

My dream in a drawing

Where I slept:

Date:

/   /

Memories from the day before

DECONSTRUCTING MY DREAM

My role in the dream:

_____

_____

_____

○ Protagonist   ○ Secondary role   ○ Not present

Other characters:

_____

_____

Feelings:

_____

_____

_____

_____

Locations / places:

_____

_____

_____

_____

Objects:

_____

_____

Sounds:

_____

_____

Genre:

○ Nightmare
○ Fantasy
○ Symbolic
○ Everyday
○ Surreal
○ Erotic

Place in time:

○ A while ago
○ Recent past
○ Present day
○ Near future
○ Distant future
○ Unknown

Type:

○ Lucid
○ Recurring
○ Unfinished
○ False awakening
○ Episodic
○ Blurry

THE STORY OF MY DREAM

CONCLUSIONS

Why I had this dream and how it can be useful to me

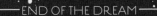
END OF THE DREAM

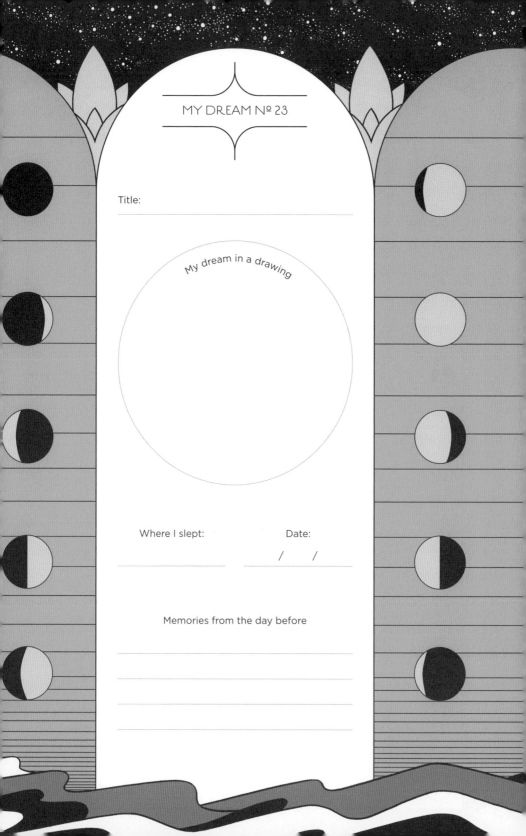

MY DREAM № 23

Title:

My dream in a drawing

Where I slept:

Date:

/   /

Memories from the day before

DECONSTRUCTING MY DREAM

My role in the dream:

_____

_____

_____

◯ Protagonist   ◯ Secondary role   ◯ Not present

Other characters:

_____

_____

Feelings:

_____

_____

_____

_____

Locations / places:

_____

_____

_____

_____

Objects:

_____

_____

Sounds:

_____

_____

Genre:

◯ Nightmare
◯ Fantasy
◯ Symbolic
◯ Everyday
◯ Surreal
◯ Erotic

Place in time:

◯ A while ago
◯ Recent past
◯ Present day
◯ Near future
◯ Distant future
◯ Unknown

Type:

◯ Lucid
◯ Recurring
◯ Unfinished
◯ False awakening
◯ Episodic
◯ Blurry

THE STORY OF MY DREAM

CONCLUSIONS

Why I had this dream and how it can be useful to me

_____
_____
_____
_____
_____
_____
_____
_____
_____
_____
_____
_____
_____
_____
_____
_____

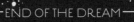

END OF THE DREAM

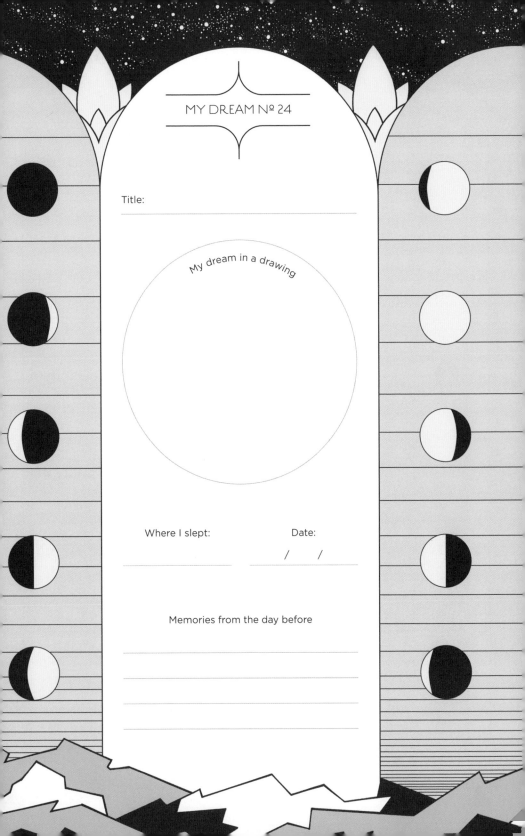

MY DREAM № 24

Title:

My dream in a drawing

Where I slept:

Date:
/   /

Memories from the day before

DECONSTRUCTING MY DREAM

My role in the dream:

_____

_____

_____

○ Protagonist   ○ Secondary role   ○ Not present

Other characters:

_____

_____

Feelings:

_____

_____

_____

_____

Locations / places:

_____

_____

_____

_____

Objects:

_____

_____

_____

Sounds:

_____

_____

_____

Genre:

○ Nightmare
○ Fantasy
○ Symbolic
○ Everyday
○ Surreal
○ Erotic

Place in time:

○ A while ago
○ Recent past
○ Present day
○ Near future
○ Distant future
○ Unknown

Type:

○ Lucid
○ Recurring
○ Unfinished
○ False awakening
○ Episodic
○ Blurry

THE STORY OF MY DREAM

CONCLUSIONS

Why I had this dream and how it can be useful to me

_____

_____

_____

_____

_____

_____

_____

_____

_____

_____

_____

_____

_____

_____

_____

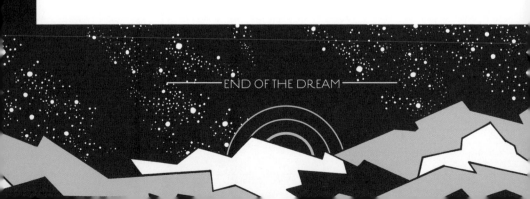

END OF THE DREAM

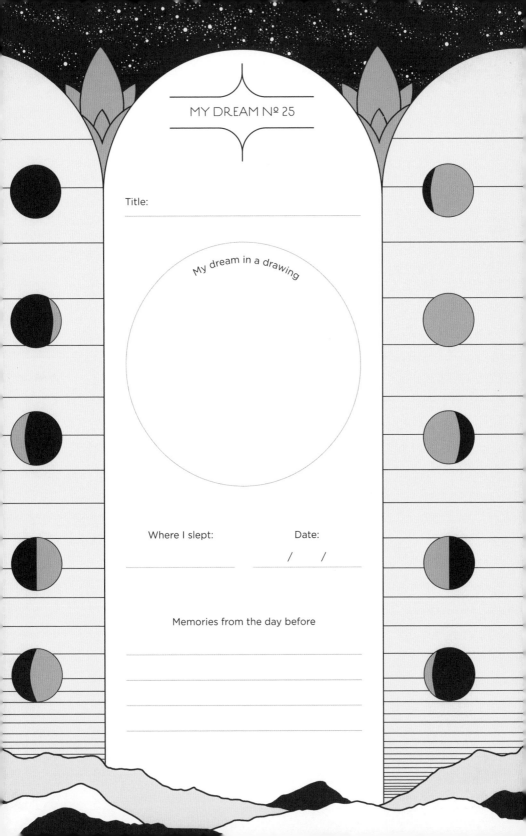

MY DREAM № 25

Title:

My dream in a drawing

Where I slept:

Date:
/   /

Memories from the day before

DECONSTRUCTING MY DREAM

My role in the dream:

_____

_____

_____

◯ Protagonist   ◯ Secondary role   ◯ Not present

Other characters:

_____

_____

Feelings:

_____

_____

_____

_____

Locations / places:

_____

_____

_____

_____

Objects:

_____

_____

Sounds:

_____

_____

Genre:

◯ Nightmare
◯ Fantasy
◯ Symbolic
◯ Everyday
◯ Surreal
◯ Erotic

Place in time:

◯ A while ago
◯ Recent past
◯ Present day
◯ Near future
◯ Distant future
◯ Unknown

Type:

◯ Lucid
◯ Recurring
◯ Unfinished
◯ False awakening
◯ Episodic
◯ Blurry

THE STORY OF MY DREAM

CONCLUSIONS

Why I had this dream and how it can be useful to me

_____

_____

_____

_____

_____

_____

_____

_____

_____

_____

_____

_____

_____

_____

_____

_____

_____

_____

_____

MY DREAM № 26

Title:
_____

My dream in a drawing

Where I slept: Date:

_____   ___/___/___

Memories from the day before

_____
_____
_____
_____

DECONSTRUCTING MY DREAM

My role in the dream:

_____

_____

_____

◯ Protagonist   ◯ Secondary role   ◯ Not present

Other characters:

_____

_____

Feelings:

_____

_____

_____

Locations / places:

_____

_____

_____

Objects:

_____

_____

Sounds:

_____

_____

Genre:

◯ Nightmare
◯ Fantasy
◯ Symbolic
◯ Everyday
◯ Surreal
◯ Erotic

Place in time:

◯ A while ago
◯ Recent past
◯ Present day
◯ Near future
◯ Distant future
◯ Unknown

Type:

◯ Lucid
◯ Recurring
◯ Unfinished
◯ False awakening
◯ Episodic
◯ Blurry

THE STORY OF MY DREAM

CONCLUSIONS

Why I had this dream and how it can be useful to me

_____

_____

_____

_____

_____

_____

_____

_____

_____

_____

_____

_____

_____

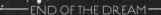

END OF THE DREAM

MY DREAM № 27

Title:
_____

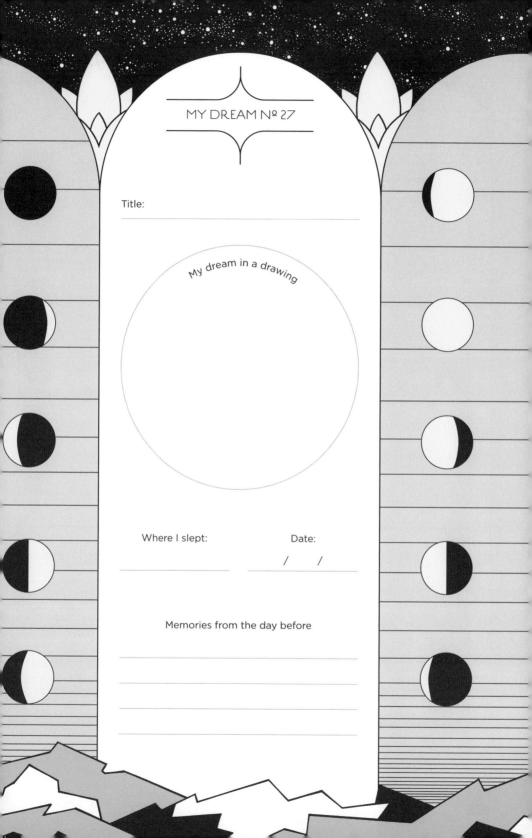

My dream in a drawing

Where I slept: Date:
                                   /   /
_____   _____

Memories from the day before

_____
_____
_____
_____

DECONSTRUCTING MY DREAM

My role in the dream:

_____

_____

_____

◯ Protagonist ◯ Secondary role ◯ Not present

Other characters:

_____

_____

Feelings:

_____

_____

_____

_____

Locations / places:

_____

_____

_____

_____

Objects:

_____

_____

Sounds:

_____

_____

Genre:

◯ Nightmare
◯ Fantasy
◯ Symbolic
◯ Everyday
◯ Surreal
◯ Erotic

Place in time:

◯ A while ago
◯ Recent past
◯ Present day
◯ Near future
◯ Distant future
◯ Unknown

Type:

◯ Lucid
◯ Recurring
◯ Unfinished
◯ False awakening
◯ Episodic
◯ Blurry

THE STORY OF MY DREAM

CONCLUSIONS

Why I had this dream and how it can be useful to me

_____

_____

_____

_____

_____

_____

_____

_____

_____

_____

_____

_____

_____

_____

_____

_____

_____

_____

_____

_____

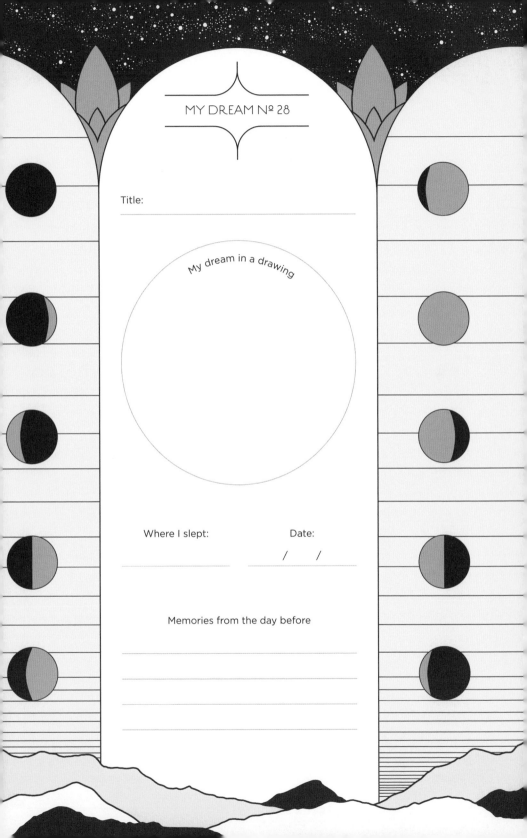

MY DREAM № 28

Title:

My dream in a drawing

Where I slept: Date:

                                  /   /

Memories from the day before

DECONSTRUCTING MY DREAM

My role in the dream:

_____

_____

_____

◯ Protagonist   ◯ Secondary role   ◯ Not present

Other characters:

_____

_____

Feelings:

_____

_____

_____

_____

Locations / places:

_____

_____

_____

_____

Objects:

_____

_____

Sounds:

_____

_____

Genre:

◯ Nightmare
◯ Fantasy
◯ Symbolic
◯ Everyday
◯ Surreal
◯ Erotic

Place in time:

◯ A while ago
◯ Recent past
◯ Present day
◯ Near future
◯ Distant future
◯ Unknown

Type:

◯ Lucid
◯ Recurring
◯ Unfinished
◯ False awakening
◯ Episodic
◯ Blurry

THE STORY OF MY DREAM

CONCLUSIONS

Why I had this dream and how it can be useful to me

_____

_____

_____

_____

_____

_____

_____

_____

_____

_____

_____

_____

_____

_____

_____

_____

_____

_____

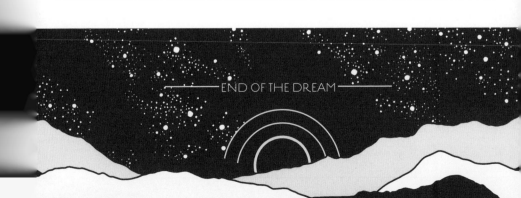

END OF THE DREAM

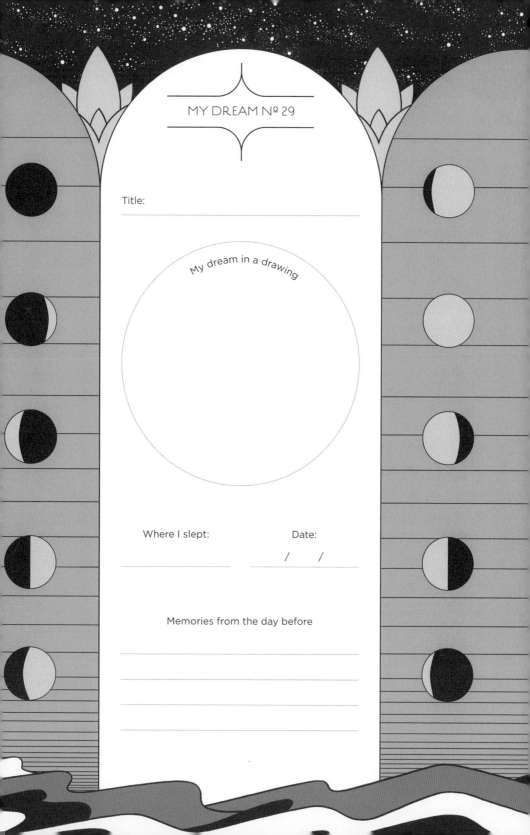

MY DREAM Nº 29

Title:

My dream in a drawing

Where I slept: Date:

/   /

Memories from the day before

DECONSTRUCTING MY DREAM

My role in the dream:

_____

_____

_____

◯ Protagonist ◯ Secondary role ◯ Not present

Other characters:

_____

_____

Feelings:

_____

_____

_____

_____

Locations / places:

_____

_____

_____

_____

Objects:

_____

_____

Sounds:

_____

_____

Genre:

◯ Nightmare
◯ Fantasy
◯ Symbolic
◯ Everyday
◯ Surreal
◯ Erotic

Place in time:

◯ A while ago
◯ Recent past
◯ Present day
◯ Near future
◯ Distant future
◯ Unknown

Type:

◯ Lucid
◯ Recurring
◯ Unfinished
◯ False awakening
◯ Episodic
◯ Blurry

THE STORY OF MY DREAM

CONCLUSIONS

Why I had this dream and how it can be useful to me

_____
_____
_____
_____
_____
_____
_____
_____
_____
_____
_____
_____
_____
_____
_____
_____

END OF THE DREAM

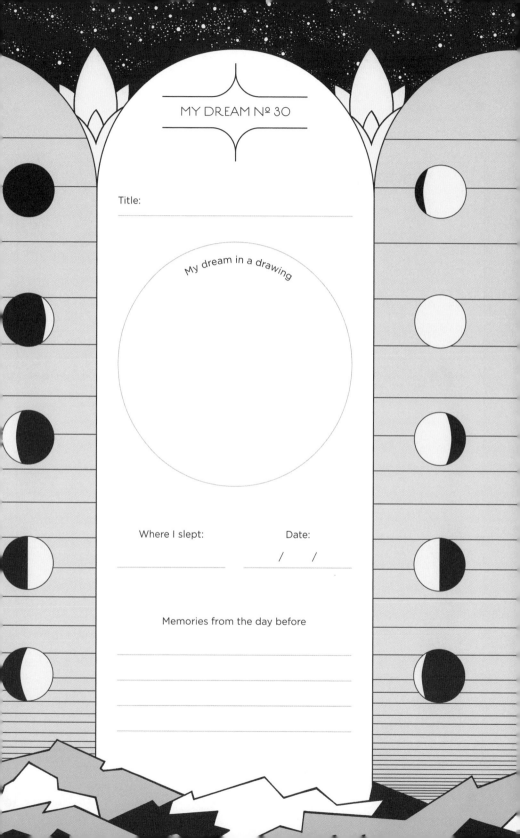

MY DREAM Nº 30

Title:

My dream in a drawing

Where I slept: Date:
                                   /   /

Memories from the day before

DECONSTRUCTING MY DREAM

My role in the dream:

_____

_____

_____

◯ Protagonist   ◯ Secondary role   ◯ Not present

Other characters:

_____

_____

Feelings:

_____

_____

_____

_____

Locations / places:

_____

_____

_____

_____

Objects:

_____

_____

Sounds:

_____

_____

Genre:

◯ Nightmare
◯ Fantasy
◯ Symbolic
◯ Everyday
◯ Surreal
◯ Erotic

Place in time:

◯ A while ago
◯ Recent past
◯ Present day
◯ Near future
◯ Distant future
◯ Unknown

Type:

◯ Lucid
◯ Recurring
◯ Unfinished
◯ False awakening
◯ Episodic
◯ Blurry

THE STORY OF MY DREAM

CONCLUSIONS

Why I had this dream and how it can be useful to me

_____

_____

_____

_____

_____

_____

_____

_____

_____

_____

_____

_____

_____

_____

_____

_____

_____

_____

—————— END OF THE DREAM ——————

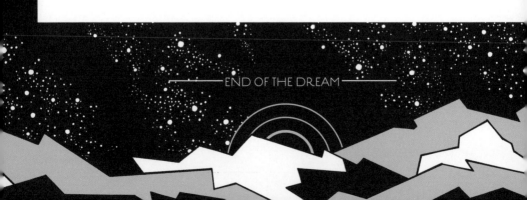

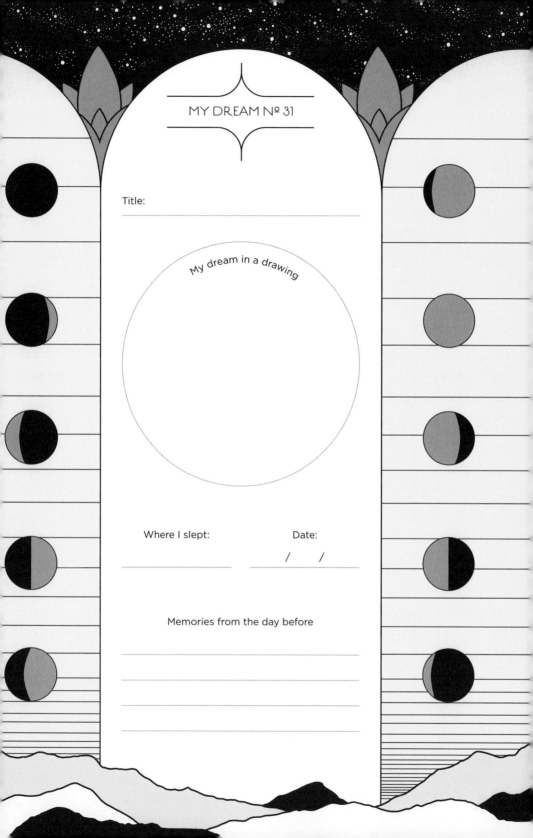

MY DREAM № 31

Title:

My dream in a drawing

Where I slept: Date:

                                    /   /

Memories from the day before

DECONSTRUCTING MY DREAM

My role in the dream:

_____

_____

_____

○ Protagonist   ○ Secondary role   ○ Not present

Other characters:

_____

_____

Feelings:

_____

_____

_____

_____

Locations / places:

_____

_____

_____

_____

Objects:

_____

_____

Sounds:

_____

_____

Genre:

○ Nightmare
○ Fantasy
○ Symbolic
○ Everyday
○ Surreal
○ Erotic

Place in time:

○ A while ago
○ Recent past
○ Present day
○ Near future
○ Distant future
○ Unknown

Type:

○ Lucid
○ Recurring
○ Unfinished
○ False awakening
○ Episodic
○ Blurry

THE STORY OF MY DREAM

CONCLUSIONS

Why I had this dream and how it can be useful to me

_____

_____

_____

_____

_____

_____

_____

_____

_____

_____

_____

_____

_____

_____

_____

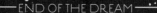

END OF THE DREAM

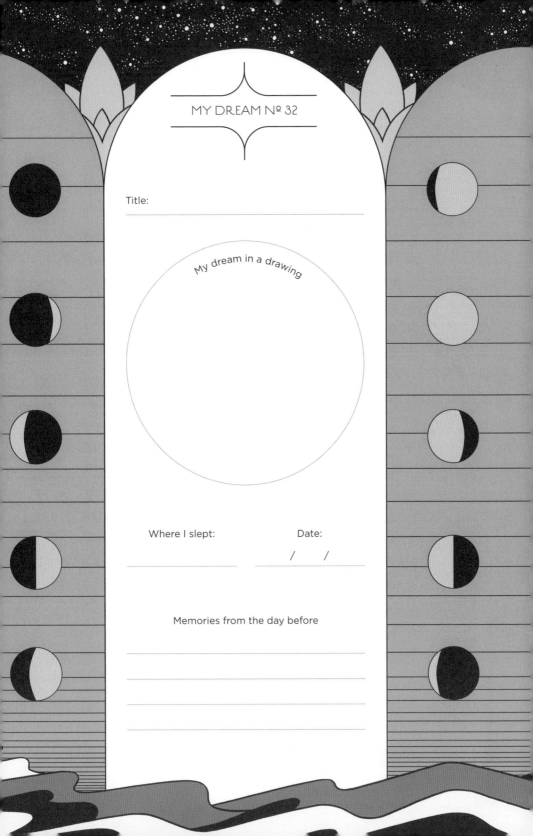

MY DREAM № 32

Title:

My dream in a drawing

Where I slept: Date:

                                        /   /

Memories from the day before

DECONSTRUCTING MY DREAM

My role in the dream:

_____

_____

_____

( ) Protagonist ( ) Secondary role ( ) Not present

Other characters:

_____

_____

Feelings:

_____

_____

_____

_____

Locations / places:

_____

_____

_____

_____

Objects:

_____

_____

Sounds:

_____

_____

Genre:

( ) Nightmare
( ) Fantasy
( ) Symbolic
( ) Everyday
( ) Surreal
( ) Erotic

Place in time:

( ) A while ago
( ) Recent past
( ) Present day
( ) Near future
( ) Distant future
( ) Unknown

Type:

( ) Lucid
( ) Recurring
( ) Unfinished
( ) False awakening
( ) Episodic
( ) Blurry

THE STORY OF MY DREAM

CONCLUSIONS

Why I had this dream and how it can be useful to me

_____

_____

_____

_____

_____

_____

_____

_____

_____

_____

_____

_____

_____

_____

_____

_____

_____

_____

_____

—————— END OF THE DREAM ——————

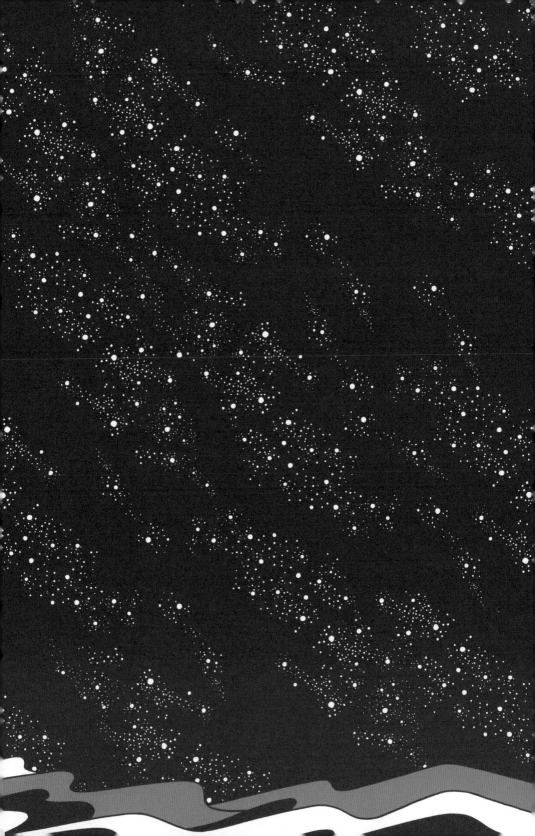

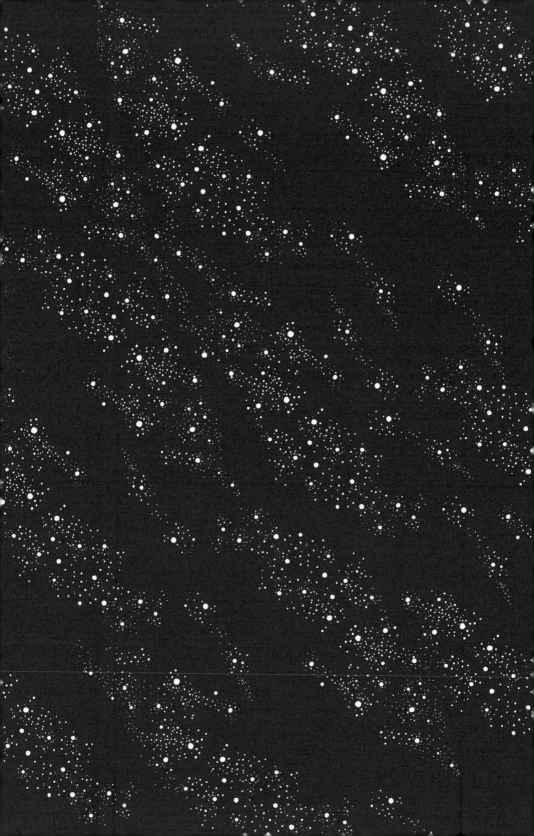

DREAMCATCHER

DREAMCATCHER

DREAMCATCHER

DREAMCATCHER

DREAMCATCHER

DREAMCATCHER

DREAMCATCHER

DREAMCATCHER

DREAMCATCHER

DREAMCATCHER

DREAMCATCHER

DREAMCATCHER

DREAMCATCHER

DREAMCATCHER

DREAMCATCHER

DREAMCATCHER

DREAMCATCHER

DREAMCATCHER

DREAMCATCHER

DREAMCATCHER

DREAMCATCHER

DREAMCATCHER

DREAMCATCHER

DREAMCATCHER

DREAMCATCHER

DREAMCATCHER

DREAMCATCHER

DREAMCATCHER

DREAMCATCHER

DREAMCATCHER

DREAMCATCHER

DREAMCATCHER

DREAMCATCHER

DREAMCATCHER

_____
_____
_____
_____
_____
_____
_____
_____
_____
_____
_____
_____
_____
_____
_____
_____
_____
_____
_____
_____
_____
_____
_____
_____
_____
_____
_____
_____
_____
_____
_____
_____

KEEP ON DREAMING

We have a lot to learn from dreams. There are exotic lands to visit, strange people to meet and powerful emotions to wrestle with every time you lie down and close your eyes. Dreams explain who we are, but also what we want, or do not want to do. We are made of the stuff of our dreams.

Who knows where our minds will take us next?